# Eat Right 4 Your Type

(REVISED AND UPDATED)

DR. PETER J. D'ADAMO

WITH CATHERINE WHITNEY

BERKLEY

NEW YORK

4 BLOOD TYPES,
4 DIETS

# Eat Right 4 Your Type

(REVISED AND UPDATED)

*The Individualized Blood Type Diet® Solution*

BERKLEY
An imprint of Penguin Random House LLC
penguinrandomhouse.com

The Library of Congress has catalogued the New American Library hardcover edition of this book as follows:

Names: D'Adamo, Peter, author. | Whitney, Catherine, author.
Title: Eat Right for Your Type: The Individualized Blood Type Diet Solution/
Dr. Peter J. D'Adamo with Catherine Whitney.
Description: Revised and updated. | New York: New American Library, [2016] |
Series: Eat Right 4 Your Type
Identifiers: LCCN 2016023719 (print) | LCCN 2016024054 (ebook) |
ISBN 9780399584169 (hardback) | ISBN 9781101042786 (ebook)
Subjects: LCSH: Blood groups. | Nutrition. | Health. | Weight loss. | Human evolution. |
BISAC: HEALTH & FITNESS/Nutrition. | HEALTH & FITNESS/Diets. |
HEALTH & FITNESS/Healthy Living.
Classification: LCC QP98 .D33 2016 (print) | LCC QP98 (ebook) |
DDC 612.1/1—dc23
LC record available at https:// lccn.loc.gov/ 2016023719

New American Library (Revised and Updated Edition) hardcover edition / December 2016
Berkley hardcover edition / September 2020

Printed in Italy by Grafica Veneta S.p.A.
11th Printing

Cover design © 1997 by Thomas Tafuri
Book design by Deborah Kerner

*To the memory of my good friend*
John J. Mosko (1919–1992)

This day is called the feast of Crispian:
He that outlives this day, and comes safe home,
Will stand a tip-toe when this day is named,
And rouse him at the name of Crispian.

AN IMPORTANT NOTE: This book is not intended as a substitute for the medical recommendations of physicians or other healthcare providers. Rather, it is intended to offer information to help the reader cooperate with physicians and health professionals in a mutual quest for optimum well-being.

The identities of people described in the case histories have been changed to protect patient confidentiality.

The publisher and the author are not responsible for any goods and/or services offered or referred to in this book and expressly disclaim all liability in connection with the fulfillment of orders for any such goods and/or services and for any damage, loss, or expense to person or property arising out of or relating to them.

# Contents

FOREWORD

# A Diet for the Twenty-First Century

The Blood Type Diet is now twenty years old. It is a happy anniversary for me and for the millions of people around the world who have bought *Eat Right for Your Type*, the book that started it all. The most striking fact about *Eat Right for Your Type* is its longevity. It's rare to see a diet book that retains its sales strength after two decades. New diets come and go every season, exploding into the marketplace only to fade before being replaced the next season by something new. And although the Blood Type Diet has often been labeled a "fad" by skeptics, the definition of *fad* is something that inspires intense fashion in the moment but quickly fades. Twenty years in, I think we can agree that the Blood Type Diet is not a fad.

In 1997, I set out to share my life's work in the first edition of this book, and frankly, I didn't know if the world would be receptive to it. At the time, most people didn't even know their blood types. They'd learned in school that blood type was important only if you needed a blood transfusion. I was proposing a radical idea: that blood type is a genetic powerhouse with a primary influence on the immune system, metabolism, and digestive processes and that different blood types have their own food preferences. Rather than being an obscure factor that you need to think about only during an emergency, knowing and understanding your blood type is actually essential to lifelong good health.

I wrote *Eat Right for Your Type* in a simple, clear fashion that every layperson could grasp. My later books would drill deeper into the scientific connections—for those interested in taking it a step further. But the goal of *Eat Right for Your Type* was to introduce the basic idea and diet. Many people were initially drawn to it because the science seemed to explain so many mysteries about their difficulties losing weight or their health complications. So they went out and got their blood typed and tried the diet. And when it worked, they told their friends, and the word spread. And spread. *Eat Right for Your Type* broke all the rules of how to be a diet book blockbuster. It wasn't an instant bestseller, but it gained momentum slowly and steadily right up to the present—with over 7 million books sold in 65 languages around the world. Its success is based not on gimmicks but on evidence and science—and results.

Long before *Eat Right for Your Type* appeared on the *New York Times* bestseller list and sold its first million copies, I could already feel that something significant was happening out there with our readers. I was inundated with emails, letters, and calls. People were emotional about their experience on the diet.

They spoke of a child's chronic ear infections suddenly gone, a mother's lifelong colitis eased, a father's symptoms of rheumatoid arthritis disappearing, a friend not needing his cholesterol or blood pressure medication anymore, and their own weight loss. They spoke of never having felt better, of having more energy, and of no longer being bloated after they ate. They spoke of medical checkups in which changes in their lab results shocked their physicians. Many of those medical doctors, along with naturopathic doctors, adopted the Blood Type Diet for their patients.

On tour speaking to groups, I was regularly approached by readers, some of them tearfully recounting how medical and fitness challenges they'd endured for years had been overcome. They often described how they had tried everything and nothing had helped them lose weight and live a healthy life until they tried the Blood Type Diet. Lifetimes of suffering were being resolved. They were getting positive results—the only measure of success that matters. And the results weren't just short-term, which is the case with most popular diets. People found the Blood Type Diet easy to follow and adopted it as a long-term way of eating and living.

This momentum kept building in spite of a huge backlash, not only from the conventional nutrition community, which had never heard of anything like this, but also from the alternative nutritional community, whose pet theories were being threatened by my methods.

I could paper my walls with all of the articles claiming that the Blood Type Diet doesn't work; most of these were based on deeply flawed studies, inexplicable rancor, or simply an intransigent attitude that something new or unknown couldn't possibly be viable. A 2014 study claiming to debunk the Blood Type Diet was particularly egregious, a study not in search of a result as much as a conclusion. After examining the study this article was based on, we found that none of the participants actually followed the diet as it was written. In one example, experimental subjects ate potato chips, sandwiches, pizza, mac-and-cheese, French fries, and processed meat products while adhering to only 13.7 percent of the guidelines and recommendations of the Blood Type Diet. The study might have debunked something, but it wasn't the Blood Type Diet.

What people in this country eat is big business. There is an institutional and financial stake in keeping the status quo alive and selling outdated concepts like the Food Pyramid or dictating universal commandments about "good" and "bad" foods. The purveyors of this misinformation are registered dietitians, health "experts," and others who have a financial and social stake in the status quo. They preach dietary wisdom as if it were delivered from the mountaintop—*meat is bad, fish is good, fat will kill you, all vegetables are healthful*—whatever the current script dictates. The one thing they don't do (and the reason the Blood Type Diet is such an outlier) is acknowledge that individuals differ, and therefore a diversity of diets makes sense. When I wrote *Eat Right for Your Type*, the word *nutrigenomics* (the way food affects gene expression) had yet to be coined, but it is a historical fact that the Blood Type Diet is the first nutrigenomic diet system. The Blood Type Diet is unique in that it presents a theory of personalized nutrition in a society where people have learned to be comfortable with a one-size-fits-all solution. However, I believe that with our growing understanding of genetics and a more sophisticated knowledge of biochemistry and gut bacteria, it's clear that personalized nutrition is the wave of the future. In this respect, the Blood Type Diet has successfully pioneered a new approach to treating people as individuals.

In the last twenty years, the scientific community has started to catch up with the fact that our blood types are critical predictive markers for disease. New studies appear every year (see Appendix G), linking blood type to yet another medical condition, and a 2016 review went so far as to say, "B group markers such as ABO and Lewis are highly promising targets for novel approaches in the field of personalized medicine." It's remarkable that while the chief tenets of the Blood Type Diet have not changed in two decades, what *has* changed is an increasing acceptance in the medical/scientific community and the population at large of the importance of blood type. The Blood Type Diet was ahead of its time, created in a period before genetic breakthroughs hit the mainstream. But the evolving understanding of biological diversity has only cemented the feasibility of this approach.

My critics still argue that the Blood Type Diet itself has not been subjected to a rigorous double-blind study, considered the gold standard for research. That might be true, but the double-blind study is a paradigm much better suited to a clean get-in, get-out trial of a single therapy or intervention, like a drug or a specific medical procedure. The logistics of testing the theory of eating according to your blood type would be staggering. Thousands of patients would have to be enrolled, their diets carefully regulated. Would people actually stick to the prescribed diet? And even if they followed it to the letter, because it takes so long for health effects to develop in people, the experiment would have to be carried out for years. What would be required to test the Blood Type Diet, a theory that involves hundreds of foods—times four, one separate test for each blood type? If the lack of a large-scale, double-blind, placebo-controlled study of the Blood Type Diet bothers you, you may also want to know that it is generally agreed that upwards of 25 percent of all prescribed pharmaceuticals lack similar proof.

That's not to say we're without evidence. Early on, I created a Blood Type Outcome Registry, where thousands of dieters documented the levels of improvement they'd experienced from their perspective, supplemented and fortified by hard data like lab tests and physician reports from those same individuals. Over the years, we've polled our many thousands of followers on social media and our website, soliciting their experiences on the Blood Type Diet. Repeatedly, our large polls have shown a level of satisfaction with the Blood Type Diet of between 85 and 90 percent. What makes this interesting is not the degree of satisfaction, because that is subjective, but rather the constancy of that number across the four blood type groups—each following a different diet specifically tailored to the requirements of that blood type.

So all I ask is that you become the study, or what we call in medicine an "N of One" (*N* is used to denote the number of participants in a research project). You have nothing to lose. Each of the four basic Blood Type Diets is healthy in its own right. Many popular diets contain similar recommendations to those found in the individual diets—the difference being they're promoted for everyone. The Blood Type Diet simply adds the extra element of knowing which of four basically healthy diets is the most healthful diet for you.

The growth of the Blood Type Diet community has been one of the most rewarding and astonishing developments of this entire journey. With the diet being adopted all over the world, it was a challenge to figure out how to reach all of these people, to offer guidance and support. Twenty years ago the Internet was in its infancy, and online communities were not very common, but we jumped in and created a simple online forum, which in time grew into an online center for educational resources, lists of targeted foods with health-promoting ingredients called nutraceuticals, supplements, training, and support that is among the most sophisticated on the web. Keeping apace with developing web opportunities, the Blood Type Diet's social media presence and smartphone app are designed to help people connect, learn, and more easily follow the diet. A groundbreaking clinic shift at the University of Bridgeport College of Naturopathic Medicine allows me to train new doctors to apply the principles of genetic individuality and the Blood Type Diet to their patients.

With millions of people following the Blood Type Diet, we thought the twentieth year was a perfect time to issue an updated version of the book. This twentieth anniversary edition of *Eat Right for Your Type* has been revised to include new information that will help people better follow the diet, along with cutting-edge research, including a new chapter on losing weight with the Blood Type Diet, edge research on blood type and the microbiome, updated disease connections, and information about tapping into the enormous worldwide support community. And if you still have your doubts, and are at all squeamish about trying the diet, the 10-Day Blood Type Diet Challenge will allow you to judge for yourself in a very short period of time whether this is the diet for you.

Looking back over the last twenty years, I experience a tremendous sense of gratitude. I started this journey as a lone voice, proposing a new way of eating and living. The science, paired with my own clinical experiences, was convincing to me, but I could never have predicted how it would take hold and grow. Thanks to the overwhelming response of the public, who trusted me and then had that trust verified, what was once labeled an odd little diet from a guy nobody had ever heard of is now a force in the nutrition world. That's how change happens.

With this edition my aim is to set the stage for the next twenty years. I invite you to join me on this fantastic voyage.

—Peter J. D'Adamo
January 2017

# Eat Right 4 Your Type

(REVISED AND UPDATED)

INTRODUCTION

# The Work of Two Lives

*I believed that no two people on the face of the earth were alike; no two people have the same fingerprints, lip prints, or voiceprints. No two blades of grass or snowflakes are alike. Because I felt that all people were different from one another, I did not think it was logical that they should eat the same foods. It became clear to me that since each person was housed in a special body with different strengths, weaknesses, and nutritional requirements, the only way to maintain health or cure illness was to accommodate to that particular patient's specific needs.*

*James D'Adamo,*
*my father*

YOUR BLOOD TYPE IS THE KEY THAT UNLOCKS THE DOOR TO THE MYSteries of health, disease, longevity, physical vitality, and emotional strength. Your blood type determines your susceptibility to illness, which foods you should eat, and how you should exercise. It is a factor in your energy levels, in the efficiency with which you burn calories, in your emotional response to stress, and perhaps even in your personality.

The connection between blood type and diet may sound radical, but it is not. We have long known that there was a missing link in our comprehension of the process that leads either to the path of wellness or to the dismal trail of disease. There had to be a reason there were so many paradoxes in dietary studies and disease survival. There also had to be an explanation for why some people were able to lose weight on particular diets, while others were not; why some people retained vitality late in life, while others deteriorated mentally and physically. Blood type analysis has given us a way to explain these paradoxes. And the more we explore the connection, the more valid it becomes.

Blood types are as fundamental as creation itself. In the masterly logic of nature, blood types follow an unbroken trail from the earliest moment of life to the present day. They are the signature of our ancient ancestors on the indestructible parchment of history.

Now we have begun to discover how to use the blood type as a cellular fingerprint that unravels many of the major mysteries surrounding our quest for good health. This work is an extension of groundbreaking findings concerning human DNA. Our understanding of blood type takes the science of genetics one step further by stating unequivocally that every human being is utterly unique. There is no right or wrong lifestyle or diet; there are only right or wrong choices to be made based on our individual genetic codes.

## How I Found the Missing Blood Type Link

MY WORK in the field of blood type analysis is the fulfillment of a lifetime pursuit—not only my own but also my father's. I am a second-generation naturopathic physician. Dr. James D'Adamo, my father, graduated from naturopathic college (a four-year postgraduate program) in 1957 and later studied in Europe at several of the great spas. He noticed that although many patients did well on strict vegetarian and low-fat diets, which are the hallmarks of "spa cuisine," a certain number of patients did not appear to improve, and some did poorly or even worsened. A sensitive man with keen powers of deduction and insight, my father reasoned that there should be some sort of blueprint that he could use to determine differences in the dietary needs of his patients. He rationalized that since blood was the fundamental source of nourishment to the body, perhaps some aspect of the blood could help identify these differences. My father set about testing this theory by blood-typing his patients and observing individualized reactions when they were prescribed different diets.

Through the years and with countless patients, a pattern began to emerge. He noticed that patients who were Type A seemed to do poorly on high-protein diets that included generous portions of meat, but did very well on vegetable proteins such as soy and tofu. Dairy products tended to produce copious amounts of mucous discharge in the sinuses and respiratory passages of Type As. When told to increase their levels of physical activity and exercise, Type A individuals usually felt fatigued and unwell; when they performed lighter forms of exercise, such as yoga, they felt alert and energized.

On the other hand, Type O patients thrived on high-protein diets, and they felt invigorated by intense physical activities, such as jogging and aerobics. The more my father tested the different blood types, the greater his conviction became that each of them followed a distinct path to wellness.

Inspired by the saying "One man's food is another man's poison," my father condensed his observations and dietary recommendations into a book he titled *One Man's Food.* When the book was published in 1980, I was in my third year of naturopathic studies at Seattle's John Bastyr College. During this time revolutionary gains were being achieved in naturopathic education. The goal of Bastyr College was nothing less than to produce the complete alternative physician, the intellectual and scientific equal of a medical internist, but with specialized naturopathic training. For the first time naturopathic techniques, procedures, and substances could be scientifically evaluated with the benefits of modern technology. I waited for an opportunity to research my father's blood type theory. I wanted to assure myself that it carried valid scientific weight. My chance came in 1982, my senior year, when, for a clinical rounds requirement, I began scanning the medical literature to see if I could find any correlation between the ABO blood types and a predilection for certain diseases, and whether any of this supported my father's diet theory. Since my father's book was based on his subjective impressions of the blood types rather than on an objective method of evaluation, I wasn't certain that I would be able to find any scientific basis for his theories. But I was amazed at what I learned.

My first breakthrough came with the discovery that two major diseases of the stomach were associated with blood type. The first was the peptic ulcer, a condition often related to higher-than-average stomach-acid levels. This condition was reported to be more common in people with Type O blood than in people with other blood types. I was immediately intrigued, since my father had observed that Type O patients did well on animal products and protein diets—foods that require more stomach acid for proper digestion.

The second correlation was an association between Type A and stomach cancer. Stomach cancer was often linked to low levels of stomach-acid production, as was pernicious anemia, another disorder found more often in Type A individuals. Pernicious anemia is related to a lack of vitamin $B_{12}$, which requires sufficient stomach acid for its absorption.

As I studied these facts I realized that on the one hand, Type O blood predisposed people to an illness associated with too much stomach acid, while on the other hand, Type A blood predisposed people to two illnesses associated with too little stomach acid.

That was the link I'd been looking for. There absolutely was a scientific basis for my father's observations. And so began my ongoing love affair with the science and anthropology of the blood types. In time, I found that my father's initial work on the correlation among blood type, diet, and health was far more significant than even he had imagined. In the coming years, scientific research would reinforce my initial findings with the publication of many studies linking blood type to nearly every metabolic and immune system condition.

My father's work has lived on in me. When he died in 2013 he was still in private practice, promoting the concepts of individualized nutrition. In one of his later writings, not long before he died, he wrote with his characteristic passion and certainty:

> *"My clarion call after practicing for 50 years is the same: all people are unique individuals, created by the shared genetics of two parents; molded by their culture, society, and geographic region in which they were raised and live; and directed by their dominant thoughts.*
>
> *"Most important, a person's blood type—whether it is O, A, B, or AB—is nature's most reliable guide in determining their individualized dietary needs."*

## Four Simple Keys to Unlock Life's Mysteries

I GREW UP in a family that was mostly Blood Type A, and because of my father's work we ate a basically Mediterranean-style diet consisting of foods such as tofu, seafood, steamed vegetables, and salads. As a child I was often embarrassed and felt somewhat deprived, because none of my friends ate weird foods like tofu. To the contrary, they were happily engaged in another kind of "diet revolution" sweeping the 1950s: their diets consisted of hamburgers, hot dogs, French fries, candy bars, ice cream, and lots of soda pop.

Today, I still eat the way I did as a child, and I love it. Every day I eat the foods that my Type A body craves, and it's immensely satisfying.

In *Eat Right for Your Type* I will teach you about the fundamental relationship between your blood type and the dietary and lifestyle choices that will help you live at your very best. The essence of the blood type connection rests in these facts:

- Your blood type—O, A, B, or AB—is a powerful genetic fingerprint in your DNA, especially when it comes to your diet.
- When you use the individualized characteristics of your blood type as a guidepost for eating and living, you will be healthier, you will naturally reach your ideal weight, and you will slow the process of aging.
- Your blood type is a more reliable measure of your identity than race, culture, or geography. It is a genetic blueprint for who you are, a guide to how you can live most healthfully.
- The key to the significance of blood type can be found in the story of human development and expansion: Type O appeared in our survivalist ancestors: hunter-gatherers; Type A evolved with agrarian society; Type B emerged as humans migrated north into colder, harsher territories; and Type AB was a thoroughly modern adaptation, a result of the intermingling of disparate groups. This evolutionary story relates directly to the dietary needs of each blood type today.

What is this remarkable factor, the blood type?

Blood type is one of several medically recognized variations, much like hair and eye color. Many of these variations, such as fingerprint patterns and DNA analyses, are used extensively by forensic scientists and criminalists as well as those who research the causes and cures of disease. Blood type is every bit as significant as other variations; in many ways, it's a more useful measure than some others. Blood type analysis is a logical system. The information is simple to learn and easy to follow. I've taught the system to numerous doctors, who tell me they are getting good results with patients who follow its guidelines. Now I will teach it to you. By learning the principles of blood type analysis, you can tailor the optimal diet for yourself and your family members. You can pinpoint the foods that make you sick, contribute to weight gain, and lead to chronic disease.

Early on, I realized that blood type analysis offered a powerful means of interpreting individual variations in health and disease. Given the amount of available research data, it is surprising that the effects of blood type on our health have not received the measure of attention that they deserve. But now I am prepared to make that information available—not just to my fellow scientists and colleagues in the medical community, but to you.

At first glance, the science of blood type may seem daunting, but I assure you it is as simple and basic as life itself. I will tell you about the ancient trail of the evolution of blood types (as riveting as the story of human history), and demystify the science of blood types to provide a clear and simple plan that you will be able to follow.

I realize that this is probably a completely new idea for you. Few people ever even think about the implications of their blood type, even though it is a powerful genetic force. The ABO gene not only controls your blood type but also affects many other processes. In particular, genes that regulate stress and digestion use ABO as a switch, turning themselves on or off depending on the specific blood type of the individual.

You may be reluctant to wade into such unfamiliar territory, even if the scientific arguments seem convincing. I ask you to do only three things: Talk to your physician before you begin, find out your blood type if you don't already know it, and try your Blood Type Diet for at least 10 days. Most of my patients experience some results within that time period—increased energy, weight loss, a lessening of digestive complaints, and improvement of chronic problems such as asthma, headaches, and heartburn. Give your Blood Type Diet a chance to bring you the benefits I've seen it bring to millions of people who swear by the diet. See for yourself that blood not only provides your body's most vital nourishment but now proves itself a vehicle for your future well-being.

# PART I

# Your Blood Type Identity

ONE

# Blood Type:

## *The Real Evolution Revolution*

BLOOD IS LIFE ITSELF. IT IS THE PRIMAL FORCE THAT FUELS the power and mystery of birth and the horrors of disease, war, and violent death. Entire civilizations have been built on blood ties. Tribes, clans, and monarchies depend on them. We cannot exist without blood—literally or figuratively.

Blood is magical. Blood is mystical. Blood is alchemic. It appears throughout human history as a profound religious and cultural symbol. Ancient peoples mixed it together and drank it to denote unity and fealty. From the earliest times, hunters performed rituals to appease the spirits of the animals they killed by offering up the animal blood and smearing it on their faces and bodies. The blood of the lamb was placed as a mark on the hovels of the enslaved Jews of Egypt so that the Angel of Death would pass over them. Moses is said to have turned the waters of Egypt to blood in his quest to free his people. The symbolic blood of Jesus Christ has been, for two thousand years, central to the most sacred rite of Christianity.

Blood evokes such rich and sacred imagery because it is in reality so extraordinary. Not only does it supply the complex delivery and defense systems that are necessary for our very existence but it provides a keystone for humanity—a looking glass through which we can trace the faint tracks of our journey.

For many decades we have been able to use biological markers such as blood type to map the movements and groupings of our ancestors. By learning how these early people adapted to the challenges posed by constantly changing climates, germs, and diets, we learn about ourselves. Change in climate and available food produced new blood types. Blood type is an unbroken cord that binds us to one another.

Ultimately, the differences in blood types reflect on the human ability to acclimate to different environmental challenges. For the most part, these challenges impacted the digestive and immune systems: a piece of bad meat could kill you; a cut or scrape could develop into a deadly infection. Yet the human race survived. And the story of that survival is inextricably tied to our digestive and immune systems. It is in these two areas that most of the distinctions between blood types are found.

## The Human Story

THE STORY OF humankind is the story of survival. More specifically, it is the story of where humans lived and what they could eat there. It is about food—about finding food and moving to find food. We don't know for certain when human evolution began. Neanderthals, the first humanoids we can recognize, may have developed 350,000 to 500,000 years ago. Maybe more.

We do know that human prehistory began in Africa, where we evolved from humanlike creatures. Early life was short, nasty, and brutish. People died a thousand different ways—opportunistic infections, parasites, animal attacks, broken bones, childbirth—and they died young.

Early humans must have had a harrowing time providing for themselves in this savage environment. Their teeth were short and blunt—ill-suited for attack. Unlike most of their competitors on the food chain, they had no special abilities in regard to speed, strength, or agility. Initially, the chief quality humans possessed was an innate cunning, which later grew to reasoned thought.

Early humans ate a rather crude diet of wild plants, grubs, and the scavenged leftovers from the kills of predatory animals. They were more prey than predator, although in time they became very accomplished hunters. Infections and parasitic afflictions were part of daily life, much more common than in our sanitized modern existence. In fact, when paleoanthropologists discover a new human coprolite (a piece of fossilized fecal waste) and analyze it in the lab, they're always amazed at the large number of parasites and worms these early people harbored within their bodies. Many of the parasites, worms, flukes, and infectious microorganisms do not stimulate the immune system to produce a specific antibody to them, a distinct advantage for Type O people because, as we will see, they already had broad protection in the form of the antibodies they carried from birth against foreign antigens. As human groups migrated into new areas, their diets changed in reaction to new environmental conditions; new food sources provoked adaptations in the digestive tract and immune system, necessary for these groups to first survive and later thrive in each new habitat. These biological changes are reflected in the remarkable differences in the worldwide distribution of the blood types, each of which appears to have flourished at critical junctures of human development.

When talking about the anthropology of the blood types it is important to distinguish between two kinds of history: molecular (gene) history and epidemiologic (population) history. Molecular history is the story of the ABO gene—the gene that determines the blood type of an individual—and this history is quite ancient. In fact the history of the ABO gene goes way beyond humans, although *Homo sapiens* (modern humans) are the only known species to possess all four ABO blood types. This is not surprising because the chemicals that make up the ABO blood types are nothing special. They can be found in everything from invertebrates to pond scum. Yet there is an important story to be told here as well. Genes are not static, and we have now begun to understand that they change and alter their function much more rapidly and dynamically than we'd previously thought possible. If you change your habits or diet, your body will turn certain genes on or off to adapt to the change, and sometimes these changes will be passed on to your offspring. This is known as the science of epigenetics.

We must also not make the mistake of thinking that, just because we share the same ABO gene with another species, the ABO gene will do the same exact things in both. For example, in certain species of pigs, having Blood Type O results in a coat of black hair. Obviously not every human who is Type O has black hair. This is because different species link a different variety of other genes to the ABO gene, a phenomenon known as *gene linkage.* As it turns out, we humans link a lot of our digestive functions to our ABO blood type rather than to our hair color.

In molecular history, the picture is a bit different. Although we can say that Type O is the oldest from the standpoint of population movement, Type A appears to be the oldest in the molecular sense, in that the mutations that gave rise to Types O and B appear to stem from it. Geneticists call this the wild-type or ancestral gene. The building blocks that make up DNA are four nucleotide bases—adenine, cytosine, guanine, thymine—referred to by the first letter of their names: A, C, G, and T. The Type B mutation is a simple replacement of one of the letters of the DNA of the ABO gene with another; what geneticists call a single nucleotide polymorphism, or SNP, pronounced *snip.* The Type O mutation is much more fascinating. It resulted from the complete loss of a letter in the ABO DNA, which is like a train that has lost a boxcar and so all the other cars just move up by one. This type of mutation is called a *frame shift* and, perhaps most amazingly, virtually every other known frame shift mutation within the genome is highly lethal. Yet if you are Type O, it *made* you.

Although Type A is the molecular ancestor, it appears to have disappeared in humans a very long time ago, and then "resurrected" itself about 300,000 years ago. This is where we now turn to the population history of blood type, and the story really starts to get interesting.

Over the last two decades I've written a lot of genomic software and have seen quite a few patients, and I can honestly tell you that spending time with people is much more interesting. Genes are an important part of the blood type story, but what your ancestors did with those genes is even more important. That is, the interactions between early humans and their environment, and how those interactions—climate, food supply, microbes and other factors—advanced the development of the blood type factors we still see today.

Much of what follows is about survival, and yes, it's the survival of the fittest. Without adequate knowledge of sanitation and zero knowledge of microbiology, our ancestors were prey to a multitude of infectious ailments. As we will explore in more detail later on in the book, there are major differences between the blood types in how individual immune systems interact with the environment. One of the most important differences involves the antibodies carried by the different blood types. These are the same antibodies that prohibit transfusing blood between certain blood types.

Now, obviously, Mother Nature did not provide us with these antibodies to mess up blood transfusion, although when talking to some physicians one can sometimes get this impression. These antibodies are part of a delicate system of defining friend from foe, self from nonself. Most authorities agree that the basic reason we have anti-other-blood-type antibodies is to act as a sort of firewall against particular germs and pathogens that just happen to also resemble the other blood types. There is compelling evidence for this. Virtually every infectious disease that afflicted our ancient ancestors has a preference for one blood type or another. Mother Nature, it seems, was merely doing what any good gambler does: hedging her bets.

Good gamblers always lead with their best card, which in this case was Type O, the simple reason being that two is a larger number than one. Type O is the only blood type with two different anti-blood-type antibodies. Type O makes anti-A, which is why it cannot take blood from Type A donors; and anti-B, which means Type B blood is a no-go as well. Although this double antibody production does limit your transfusion options, it also produces a form of broad-spectrum immune protection. With its better immune protection Type O got the jump on the other blood types—including Type A, which, as I mentioned, it mutated from—and as the dictator Joseph Stalin is said to have observed, "Quantity has a quality all its own."

In this context, the story of blood type can be summarized this way:

1. Survival, expansion, and ascent of humans to the top of the food chain (Type O to its fullest expression).
2. The change from hunter-gatherer to a more domesticated agrarian lifestyle (advance of the original Type A).

3. The merging and migration of population groups from the African homeland to Europe, Asia, and the Americas (advance of Type B).
4. The modern intermingling of disparate groups (the arrival of Type AB).

Each blood type contains the genetic message of our ancestors' diets and behaviors, and though we're a long way away from early history, many of their traits still affect us. Knowing these predispositions helps us understand the logic of the Blood Type Diet.

## O Is for Old

MODERN HUMANS may have emerged out of Africa as recently as 60,000 years ago, although other ancestral humans were certainly well distributed throughout Asia and Europe by that time and had developed hunter-gatherer type technologies and the ability to control fire. At about this same time it is thought that humans developed the phonetic diversity necessary for true speech and communication. These skills propelled the human species to the top of the food chain, making them the most dangerous predators on earth. They began to hunt in organized packs; in a short time, they were able to make improved weapons and advanced tools. These major developments gave them strength and superiority beyond their natural physical abilities.

Skillful and formidable hunters, the early modern humans soon had little to fear from any of their animal rivals. With no natural predators other than themselves, the population exploded. Protein—meat—was their fuel, and it was probably at this point that gene followed function. Besides its double-barreled antibody armory there is one other observation that indicates that we are by and large talking about Type O during this period.

In the 1940s and 1950s the geneticist Arthur Mourant studied the distribution of the ABO blood types across the globe. What made Mourant's work so important was that he studied the blood type distributions of indigenous peoples. Studying blood type distributions in modern populations would be essentially useless, as over the last millennia humans have intermingled to a very great degree.

Mourant's findings were very interesting. In virtually every society where an indigenous population (such as the Inuits or Native Americans) was isolated or otherwise separated from contact with other groups over a long period of time the percentage of Blood Type O skyrocketed, at times reaching over 90 percent of the total population. And all of these populations, where still possible, pursued a hunter-gatherer type of existence.

Genes can alter their function based on changes in the environment: change a habit for long enough and the body will alter the functions of genes needed to metabolize the result of that change. As we will soon see, Type Os possess many of the digestive characteristics needed to make an effective hunter-gatherer.

These early humans thrived on meat, and it took a remarkably short time for them to kill off the big game within their hunting range. Evidence suggests that these Paleolithic hunters were quite healthy: bone fossils indicate that they were taller than their ancestors. This may have led to an explosion in the population, a persistent problem

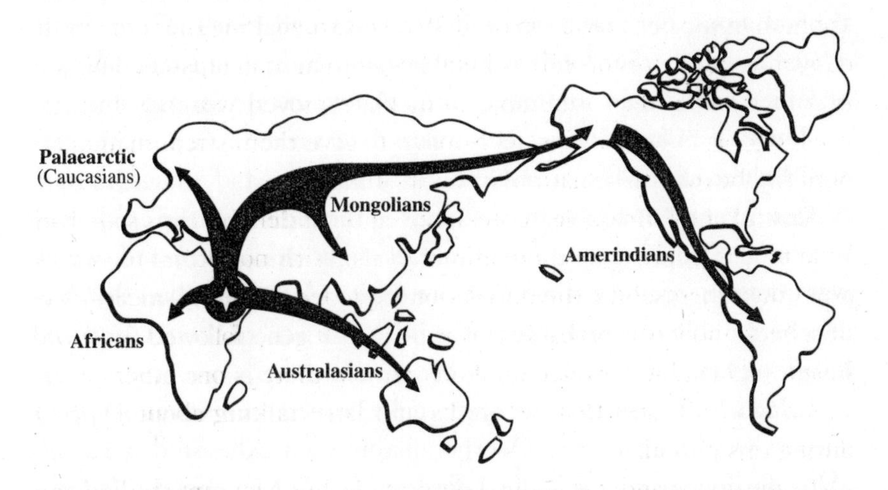


*From their base in the ancestral homeland of Africa, early Blood Type O hunter-gatherers wandered throughout Africa and into Europe and Asia in search of new supplies of large game. As they encountered changing environmental conditions, they began to develop modern physical and physiological characteristics.*

for hunter-gatherer societies. More mouths to feed and dwindling game reserves prompts migration.

Migration often leads to conflict, especially if you are the person who already occupies the land others are migrating to. Hunters began fighting and killing others who were impinging on what they claimed were their exclusive hunting grounds. As always, human beings found their greatest enemy to be themselves. Good hunting areas became scarce. The migration of the human race began.

Bands of hunters were traveling farther and farther in search of meat. When a shift in the trade winds desiccated what had been fertile hunting land in the African Sahara, and when previously frozen northern areas grew warmer, people began to move out of Africa into Europe and Asia.

This movement seeded the planet with its base population, which was Blood Type O, the numerically predominant blood type even today.

By 20,000 B.C.E. modern humans had moved fully into Europe and Asia, decimating the vast herds of large game to such an extent that other foods had to be found. Searching each new area for anything edible, it is likely that humans quickly became omnivorous, with a mixed diet of berries, grubs, nuts, roots, and small animals. Populations also thrived along the coastlines and the lakes and rivers of the earth, where fish and other foods were abundant. By 10,000 B.C.E., humans occupied every main landmass on the planet, except for Antarctica.

The movement of the early humans to less temperate climates created lighter skins, less massive bone structures, and straighter hair. Nature, over time, acclimated humans to the regions of the earth they inhabited. People moved northward, so light skin developed, which was better protected against frostbite than dark skin. Lighter skin was also better able to metabolize vitamin D in a land of shorter days and longer nights.

Paleolithic hunter-gatherers eventually burned themselves out; their success was an anathema. Overpopulation soon exhausted the available hunting grounds. What had once seemed like an unending supply of large game animals diminished sharply. This led to increased competition for the remaining hunting grounds. Competition led to war, and war to further migration.

It is interesting to note that almost every society carried down in its history a story of creation that involved an early time of paradise followed by an eventual downfall and expulsion. Many experts in the field of folklore believe that these stories all stem from a distant memory of a halcyon time of freedom and abundance, followed by a time of shortage and struggle. It you are Type O, that memory of paradise is locked into your genetic memory.

## A Is for Agrarian

THE PERIOD between the decline of Paleolithic existence and the advent of agricultural technology is not very well-defined. However, much like the man with one foot in his boat and one foot on the dock, we can conclude that this intermediate period was somewhat precarious. We can assume a certain hardscrabble, hand-to-mouth existence was the order of the day, perhaps not unlike what we still see to this day in areas of famine. When hungry we will eat, or attempt to eat, almost anything.

However, somewhere in Asia or the Middle East between 25,000 and 15,000 B.C.E. humans began to understand that plant energy could be controlled, and even optimized. This is the beginning of the so-called Neolithic Revolution, with its hallmarks of agriculture and animal domestication. This new technology probably started with a strain of notoriously bitter legumes known as vetches, and moved on to different grains, which in fact started out in nature as simple wild grasses.

As anyone with hay fever can tell you, grasses are among the most allergy-inducing things in nature. In fact, plant food products are typically more allergenic than animal foods. This is a dilemma for the immune system: how can one derive nutrients from foods that also induce allergic reactions? The solution, as in many other dilemmas, is tolerance.

Good design is, in a way, a form of negotiation, and a good negotiation is usually defined as resulting in both parties leaving the table mildly dissatisfied with the final result. If you study the physiology of Blood Type A, it soon appears evident that this is a blood type that tries mightily to get along with others, often perhaps to a fault, as we will soon see.

The cultivation of grains changed everything. Unlike animal proteins, which require a simple, yet powerful, mix of stomach acid and protein-digestion enzymes, plant proteins require a slower, more nuanced approach. You have to first figure out how to render them innocuous to the immune system before you can move on to metabolizing them. Able to forgo their hand-to-mouth existence and sustain themselves for the first time, people established stable communities and permanent living structures. This radically different lifestyle, a major change in diet and environment, resulted in the need for entirely new characteristics in the digestive tracts and immune systems of the Neolithic peoples—changes that allowed them to better tolerate and absorb cultivated grains and other agricultural products. Type A was in the spotlight. Evidence clearly indicates that the advance of farming technology geographically parallels the distribution of Blood Type A in ancient populations.

Settling into permanent farming communities presented new developmental challenges. The skills necessary for hunting together now gave way to a different kind of cooperative society. Agriculture could allow for an almost infinite increase in population and for specialization and division of labor. For the first time, a specific skill at doing one thing depended on the skills of others doing something else. For example, the miller depended on the farmer to bring in crops; the farmer depended on the miller to grind the grain. One no longer thought of food as only an immediate source of nourishment or as a sometime thing. Fields needed to be sown and cultivated in anticipation of future reward. Planning and networking with others became the order of the day. Psychologically, these are traits at which Type As excel—perhaps another environmental adaptation.

Agriculture also required the concentration of resources, leading to the beginning of urban existence. This is again reflected in the distribution of blood type on the world map. Mourant's maps clearly show a high percentage of Blood Type A in the areas of the world with long histories of urban living.

What could have been the reason for this extraordinary rate of growth in the number of Type A individuals? It was survival. Survival of the fittest in a crowded society. Because Type A emerged as more resistant to infections common to densely populated areas, urban industrialized societies quickly became Type A. Even today, survivors of plague and cholera show a predominance of Type A over Type O.

Eventually, the gene for Type A blood spread beyond Asia and the Middle East into Western Europe, carried by people such as the Indo-Europeans, a seminomadic people who penetrated deeply into the pre-Neolithic populations and gave us the foundation for most of our modern languages.

Today, Type A blood is still found in its highest concentration among Western Europeans. The frequency of Type A diminishes as we head eastward through Europe, following the receding trails of the ancient migratory patterns. Type A people are highly concentrated across the Mediterranean, Adriatic, and Aegean seas, particularly in Corsica, Sardinia, Spain, Turkey, and the Balkans. The Japanese also have some of the highest concentrations of Type A blood in eastern Asia, along with a moderately high number of Type B.

Blood Type A surged in response to the dietary changes stemming from the conversion of the Paleolithic hunter-gatherer way of life into the Neolithic urban-agricultural revolution, including the changes in diet and the exposure to new diseases that this lifestyle brought with it. It was almost as if Mother Nature were presenting us with a signpost at a fork in the road as well as a source for innumerable diet controversies: Paleo/high-protein diet to the left, Asian/Mediterranean diet to the right. Two powerful enough formulas by the standards of your typical one-size-fits-all diet book. But, as it turns out, the story of blood type is even richer and more sophisticated.

## B Is for Balance

Blood Type B appears to have reached significant numbers sometime between 10,000 and 15,000 B.C.E., in the area of the Himalayan highlands—now part of present-day Pakistan and India—where it may have initially developed its characteristics in response to climatic changes. It is interesting that many of its physiological characteristics appear to vary with altitude: Studies show that women who are Type B are taller and get their menses earlier the higher up they live.

Of all the ABO blood types, Type B has the most unusual and specific distribution on the world map: a huge swath of territory extending north to south right across the area where Europe meets Asia. Type B is found in increased numbers from Japan, Mongolia, China, and India up to the Ural Mountains. From there westward, the percentages fall until a low is reached at the western tip of Europe.

This was traditionally an area that was home to a mix of Caucasian and Mongolian tribes, and Type B is very characteristic of the great tribes of steppe-dwellers, who once dominated the Eurasian plains.

As the steppe-dwellers swept through Asia, the gene for Type B blood was spread along the way. The groups ranged northward, pursuing a culture dependent on herding and domesticating animals—as their diet of meat and cultured dairy products reflected.

Two distinct groups of Type B sprang up as the pastoral nomads pushed into Asia: an agrarian, comparatively sedentary group in the south and the east, and a nomadic, warlike society conquering the north and the west. The nomads were expert horsemen who penetrated far into eastern Europe: Like a wave at the seashore, Type B blood can be found in many eastern European populations, but dissipates rapidly the farther west we look.

A study of blood group patterns in the United Kingdom showed that Blood Type B, although not common there, was found to be in great concentration along the internal rivers, indicating a path of invasion by and/or commerce with Norsemen who had perhaps picked it up from their raids into present-day Russia.

In the meantime, an entire agriculturally based culture had spread throughout China and Southeast Asia. Because of the nature of the land they chose to till and the climates unique to their areas, these people created and employed sophisticated irrigation and cultivation techniques that displayed an awesome blend of creativity, intelligence, and engineering.

The schism between the warlike tribes to the north and the peaceful farmers to the south was deep, and its remnants exist to this day in southern Asian cuisine, which consists of little if any dairy foods. To many Asian minds, dairy products are the food of the barbarian, which is unfortunate because the diet they have adopted does not suit their Type B blood as well.

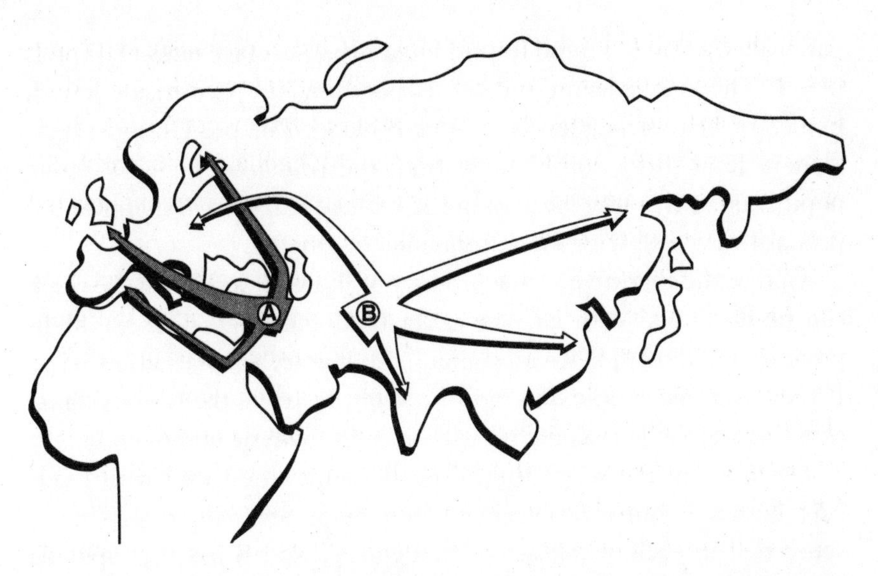


*Origins and movements of Type A and Type B. From its beginnings in Asia and the Middle East, the gene for Type A was carried by Indo-European peoples into western and northern Europe. Other migrations carried Type A into northern Africa, where it spread into the Saharan populations. From its origins in the western Himalayan mountains, Type B was carried by Mongolian peoples into southeast Asia and into the Asian flatlands, or steppes. A separate migration of Type B people entered eastern Europe. By this time, sea levels had risen, removing the land bridge between North America and Asia. This prevented any movement of Type B into North America, where the Native American populations continued on as exclusively Type O.*

---

The small numbers of Type B individuals among old and western Europeans represents western migration by Asian nomadic peoples. This is best seen in the east-central Europeans—the Germans and Austrians—who have an unexpectedly high incidence of Type B blood compared to their western neighbors. The highest occurrence of Type B in Germans occurs in the area around the upper and middle Elbe River, which had been nominally held as the dividing line between civilization and barbarism in ancient times.

Modern subcontinental Indians, a Caucasian people, have some of the highest frequencies of Type B blood in the world. The northern Chinese and Koreans have very high rates of Type B blood and very low rates of Type A.

The blood type characteristics of Jewish populations have long been of interest to anthropologists. As a general rule, regardless of their nationality, there is a trend toward higher-than-average rates of Type B blood. The Ashkenazim and the Sephardim, the two major Jewish branches, share strong levels of Type B blood. The pre-Diaspora Babylonian Jews differ considerably from the primarily Type O Arabic population of Iraq (the location of the biblical Babylon) in that they are primarily Type B, with some frequency of Type A.

Unlike the digestive characteristics of Type O and Type A, which can be described with easy-to-understand concepts, such as "high-protein diet" and "plant-based diet," the dietary adaptations of Type B seem to resist simple description. Over the years, the best explanation I've been able to come up with is "idiosyncratic omnivore."

*Omnivore* in the sense that Type B seems to do well with foods from both the animal and vegetable kingdoms, and *idiosyncratic* in the sense that in each of these food categories Type B has very specific strengths and weaknesses that are experienced only by those who are Type B. Many of the relationships seem to defy logic—such as the notion that chicken is a problem food, while turkey is not, although, for most of us, there would appear to be little difference between the two. We'll explore these fascinating relationships when we introduce the concept of food lectins later in the book.

## AB Is for Modern

IN GENETICS it appears that blood type plays by its own rules. As we've seen with Type O, you can have what is normally a lethal mutation and simply wind up with a different blood type. With Type A you can have an ancient gene that, for some unknown reason, decided to exit the stage eons ago and then resurrect itself. With Type B your physiology appears to change as you change altitude. However, with Type AB, Mother Nature may have saved the best for last.

Like most genes, ABO blood type exists in a sort of dominant–submissive relationship. Certain variations, known as alleles, are just stronger than others. For example, given an allele for brown eyes from one parent and an allele for blue eyes from another, you will most likely wind up with brown eyes. Brown eyes are the dominant trait and blue eyes the submissive, or recessive, trait.

Of course, blood type genetics works things out in a unique way. Like other genes, there are dominant alleles (A and B) and a submissive one (O), and from here the math is rather simple: If you receive either a B allele or an A allele from one parent and an O allele from the other, you'll be either Type A or Type B. You can be Type O only if both parents give you an O allele. But because the recessive O is more common than either A or B, there are more Type O individuals in the population.

But what happens if one parent gives you an A allele and the other a B allele? The obvious answer (which is in fact true) is that you become Blood Type AB. But like any good puzzle, it is the *why* that is the most interesting part.

Just like the mutation that creates Type O breaks all the rules for the average mutation, how a person gets to be Type AB turns out to be another rule breaker. In genetic parlance (and the criteria for any good relationship), the A allele and B allele are said to be *co-dominant.* That is, they simply co-exist with each other.

Thus we arrive at the basic essence of Type AB: It is not an adaptation in the sense that the development of O, A, and B were adaptations to climate, diet and disease. Instead, it came into being through the simple circumstance of a population of Type A blood colliding and cohabitating with a population of Type B blood. You might think this is nothing special, but remember our earlier discussions—for a long, long time, Type A resided in one part of the globe, and Type B in a different part. It has only been in the last 1,000 to maybe 2,000 years that there was any kind of real interaction between the two.

Until ten or twelve centuries ago, there was no Type AB blood. Then barbarian hordes sliced through the soft underbelly of many collapsing civilizations, overrunning the length and breadth of the Roman Empire. As a result of the intermingling of these eastern invaders with the last trembling vestiges of ancient European civilization, Type AB blood came to be. No evidence for the occurrence of this blood type extends beyond that time, when a large western migration of eastern peoples took place. Blood Type AB is rarely found in European graves before 900 C.E. Studies on exhumations of prehistoric graves in Hungary show a distinct lack of Type AB into the fourth to seventh century C.E. This would seem to indicate that up until that point in time, European populations of Type A and Type B did not come into common contact, or if so, rarely mingled or intermarried.

Because Type ABs inherit the tolerance of both Type A and Type B, their immune system has an enhanced ability to manufacture more specific antibodies to microbial infections. This unique quality of possessing neither anti-A nor anti-B antibodies minimizes the chances of being prone to allergies and other autoimmune diseases such as arthritis, inflammation, and lupus. There is, however, a greater predisposition to certain cancers because Type AB responds to anything A-like or B-like as "self," so it manufactures no opposing antibodies.

Type AB presents a multifaceted, and sometimes perplexing, blood type identity. It is the first blood type to adopt an amalgamation of immune characteristics, some of which make it stronger, and some of which are in conflict. Perhaps Type AB presents the perfect metaphor for modern life: complex and unsettled.

## The Blending Grounds

BLOOD TYPE, geography, and race are woven together to form our human identity. We may have cultural differences, but when you look at blood type, you see how superficial they are. Your blood type is older than your ethnicity and more fundamental than your nationality. The blood types were not a hit-or-miss act of random genetic activity. Each blood type developed as an adaptation to a series of cataclysmic chain reactions, spread over eons of environmental upheaval and change—dietary, environmental, and geographical—that became part of the evolutionary engine that ultimately produced the different characteristics of each blood type.

Some anthropologists believe that classifying humans into races invites oversimplification. Blood type is a far more important determinant of individuality and similarity than is race. For example, an African and a European of Type A blood could exchange blood or organs and have many of the same aptitudes, digestive functions, and immunological structures—characteristics they would not share with a member of their own ethnic group or nationality who was Blood Type B.

Racial distinctions based on skin colors, ethnic practices, geographical homelands, or cultural roots are not a valid way to distinguish among people. Members of the human race have a lot more in common with one another than we may have ever suspected. We are all potentially brothers and sisters. In blood.

Today, as we look back on this remarkable evolutionary revolution, it is clear that our ancestors had unique biological blueprints that complemented their environments. It is this lesson we bring with us into our current understanding of blood types, for the genetic characteristics of our ancestors live in our blood today.

- TYPE O: The most widespread early mutation and most basic blood type, the survivor at the top of the food chain, with a strong and ornery immune system willing to and capable of destroying anyone, friend or foe.
- TYPE A: The first adaptors, forced by the necessity of migration and shortage to adapt to a more agrarian diet and lifestyle.
- TYPE B: The assimilator, the idiosyncratic omnivore, adapting to new climates and the mingling of populations.
- TYPE AB: The enigma, the unique offspring of a rare merger between the opposing forces of tolerance and adaptation.

Our ancestors left each of us a special legacy, imprinted in our blood types. This legacy exists permanently in the nucleus of each cell. It is here that the anthropology and science of our blood meet.

TWO

# Blood Code:

## *The Blueprint of Blood Type*

BLOOD IS A FORCE OF NATURE, THE ÉLAN VITAL THAT HAS SUSTAINED us since time immemorial. A single drop of blood, too small to see with the naked eye, contains the entire genetic code of a human being. The DNA blueprint is intact and replicated within us endlessly—through our blood.

Our blood also contains eons of genetic memory—bits and pieces of specific programming, passed on from our ancestors in codes we are still attempting to comprehend. A crucial part of this code rests within our blood type. Perhaps it is the most important code we can decipher in our attempt to unravel the mysteries of blood and its vital role in our existence.

To the naked eye, blood is a homogeneous red liquid. But under the microscope, blood shows itself to be composed of many different elements. The abundant red blood cells contain a special type of iron that our bodies use to carry oxygen and create the blood's characteristic rust color. White blood cells, far less numerous than red, cruise our bloodstreams like ever-vigilant troops, protecting us against infection.

This complex living fluid also contains proteins that deliver nutrients to the tissues, platelets that help it clot, and plasma that contains the guardians of our immune system.

## The Importance of Blood Type

You may be unaware of your own blood type unless you've donated blood or needed a transfusion. Most people think of blood type as an inert factor, something that comes into play only when there is a hospital emergency. But now that you have heard the dramatic story of the roots of blood type, you are beginning to understand that blood type has always been the driving force behind human survival, changing and adapting to new conditions, environments, and food supplies.

Why is our blood type so powerful? What is the essential role it plays in our survival—not just thousands of years in the past, but today?

Your blood type is the key to your body's entire immune system. It controls the influence of viruses, bacteria, infections, chemicals, stress, and the entire assortment of invaders and conditions that might compromise your immune system.

The word *immune* comes from the Latin *immunis*, which denoted a city in the Roman Empire that was not required to pay taxes. (If only your blood type could give you that kind of immunity!) The immune system works to define "self" and destroy "non-self." This is a critical function, for without it your immune system could attack your own tissues by mistake or allow a dangerous organism access to vital areas of your body. In spite of all its complexity, the immune system boils down to two basic functions: recognizing "us" and killing "them." In this respect your body is like a large invitation-only party. If the prospective guest supplies the correct invitation, the security guards allow her to enter and enjoy herself. If an invitation is lacking or forged, the guest is forcibly removed.

## Enter the Blood Type

Nature has endowed our immune system with very sophisticated methods to determine if a substance in the body is foreign or not. One method involves chemical markers called *antigens*, which are found on the cells of our bodies. Every life-form, from the simplest virus to humans themselves, has unique antigens that form a part of its chemical fingerprint. One of the most powerful antigens in the human body is the one that determines your blood type. The different blood type antigens are so sensitive that when they are operating effectively, they are the immune system's greatest security system. When your immune system sizes up a suspicious character (that is, a foreign antigen) one of the first things it looks for is your blood type antigen to tell it whether the intruder is friend or foe.

Each blood type possesses a different antigen with its own special chemical structure. Your blood type is named for the blood type antigen you possess on your red blood cells.

| IF YOU ARE | YOU HAVE THIS ANTIGEN ON YOUR CELLS |
|---|---|
| BLOOD TYPE A | A |
| BLOOD TYPE B | B |
| BLOOD TYPE AB | A AND B |
| BLOOD TYPE O | NO ANTIGENS |

Visualize the chemical structure of blood types as antennae of sorts, projecting outward from the surface of our cells into deep space. These antennae are made from long chains of a repeating sugar called fucose, which by itself forms the simplest of the blood types, Blood Type O. The early discoverers of blood type called it "O" as a way to make us think of "zero" or "no real antigen." This antenna also serves as the base for the other Blood Types, A, B, and AB.

- BLOOD TYPE A is formed when the O antigen, or fucose, plus another sugar called *N*-acetyl-galactosamine, is added. So fucose plus *N*-acetyl-galactosamine equals Blood Type A.
- BLOOD TYPE B is also based on the O antigen, or fucose, but has a different sugar, named D-galactosamine, added on. So fucose plus D-galactosamine equals Blood Type B.
- BLOOD TYPE AB is based on the O antigen, fucose, plus the two sugars, *N*-acetyl-galactosamine and D-galactosamine. So fucose plus *N*-acetyl-galactosamine plus D-galactosamine equals Blood Type AB.

**The Four Blood Types and Their Antigens**

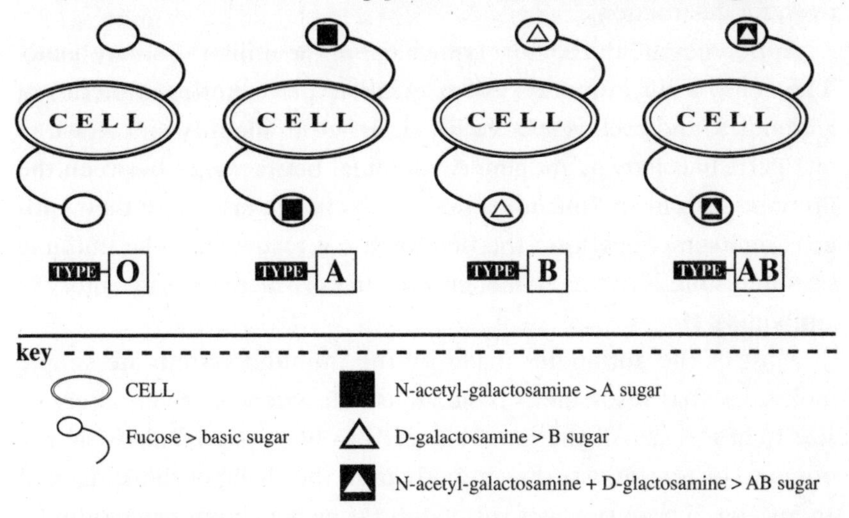


*The four blood types and their antigens. Type O is the stalk, fucose; Type A is fucose plus the sugar* N*-acetyl-galactosamine; Type B is fucose plus the sugar* D*-galactosamine; Type AB is fucose plus the A sugar and the B sugar.*

At this point you may be wondering about other blood type identifiers, such as positive and negative. Usually, when people tell their blood types they say, "I'm A positive." Or "I'm O negative." These variations, or minor blood types, play relatively insignificant roles. More than 90 percent of all the factors associated with your blood type are related to your primary type—O, A, B, or AB. However, one additional influence, secretor status, can be important, and we'll describe it later. For now we will concentrate on your ABO blood type itself.

## Antigens Create Antibodies (Immune System Smart Bombs)

WHEN YOUR IMMUNE SYSTEM SENSES that a foreign antigen has entered the system, the first thing it does is create antibodies to that antigen. These antibodies, specialized chemicals manufactured by the cells of the immune system, are designed to attach to and tag the foreign antigen for destruction.

Antibodies are the cellular equivalent of the military's smart bomb. The cells of our immune system manufacture countless varieties of antibodies, and each is specifically designed to identify and attach to one particular foreign antigen. A continual battle wages between the immune system and intruders that try to change or mutate their antigens into some new form the body will not recognize. The immune system responds to this challenge with an ever-increasing inventory of antibodies.

Most of the antibodies made by the immune system are simple molecules that resemble a basic adjustable wrench, which alters its size to fit the size of the nut that needs to be twisted. Likewise, the immune system adjusts the antibody to fit the shape of the antigen of an invader. These types of antibodies (known as immunoglobulin G, or IgG) simply tag the foreign object. The combination of the invader and this type of antibody alerts the patrolling cells of the immune system, which move to the invader, attach to the antibody, and attack and destroy it.

However, the antibodies that we make as part of our ABO blood type are different. These antibodies (known as IgM) are very large molecules that resemble a snowflake; they have multiple attachment points and are made without stimulation of the immune system. When they encounter an antigen that resembles an opposing blood type, they change their form from a snowflake to something resembling a crab. This allows them to produce a reaction called agglutination (literally, "gluing"). This type of crablike antibody attaches to the foreign antigen and makes it very sticky. When cells, viruses, parasites, and bacteria are agglutinated, they stick together and clump up, which makes it easier for the body to dispose of them. This is why getting a transfusion of the wrong blood type is so deadly. The antibodies you have against the wrong blood type attack the transfused blood and trigger massive agglutination, which leads to shock and possibly death.

The anti-other-blood-type antibodies are the strongest antibodies in our immune system, and their ability to clump—agglutinate—the blood cells of a different blood type is so powerful that it can be immediately observed on a glass slide with the unaided eye. Most of our other antibodies require some sort of stimulation (such as a vaccination or an infection) for their production. The blood type antibodies are different: They are produced automatically, often appearing at birth and reaching almost adult levels by four months of age. Evidence suggests that they are stimulated by the first bacteria that begin to inhabit the newborn's gut and, perhaps not surprising, by the first foods they eat.

As microbes must rely on their slippery powers of evasion, this agglutination is a very powerful defense mechanism. It is rather like handcuffing criminals together; they become far less dangerous than when they are allowed to move around freely. Sweeping the body for odd cells, viruses, parasites, and bacteria, the antibodies herd the undesirables together for easy identification and disposal.

The system of blood type antigens and antibodies has other ramifications besides detecting microbial and other invaders. More than a hundred years ago, Karl Landsteiner, a brilliant Austrian physician and scientist, also found that blood types produced antibodies to other blood types. His revolutionary discovery explained why some people could exchange blood, while others could not. Until Landsteiner's time, blood transfusions were a hit-or-miss affair. Sometimes they "took," and sometimes they didn't, and nobody knew why. Thanks to Landsteiner, we now know which blood types are recognized as friend by other blood types, and which are recognized as foe.

Landsteiner learned that

- Blood Type A carries anti-B antibodies. Type B is rejected by Type A.
- Blood Type B carries anti-A antibodies. Type A is rejected by Type B.

Thus Type A and Type B cannot exchange blood.

- Blood Type AB carries no antibodies. The universal receiver, it accepts any other blood type. But because it carries both A and B antigens, it is rejected by all other blood types.

Thus Type AB can receive blood from everyone, but can give blood to no one. Except another Type AB, of course.

- BLOOD TYPE O carries anti-A and anti-B antibodies. Type A, Type B, and Type AB are rejected.

Thus Type O can't receive blood from anyone but another Type O. But free of A and B antigens, Type O can give blood to everyone else. Type O is the universal donor.

| IF YOU ARE | YOU CARRY ANTIBODIES AGAINST |
|---|---|
| BLOOD TYPE A | BLOOD TYPE B |
| BLOOD TYPE B | BLOOD TYPE A |
| BLOOD TYPE AB | NO ANTIBODIES |
| BLOOD TYPE O | BLOOD TYPES A AND B |

But there is much more to the agglutination story. It was also found that many foods agglutinate the cells of certain blood types (in a way similar to rejection) but not others, meaning a food that may be harmful to the cells of one blood type may be beneficial to the cells of another. It's not surprising that many of the antigens in these foods have A-like or B-like characteristics. This discovery provided an entirely different scientific link between blood type and diet. Remarkably, however, its revolutionary implications would lie dormant, gathering dust for most of the twentieth century—until a handful of scientists, doctors, and nutritionists began to explore the connection.

## Lectins: The Diet Connection

A CHEMICAL REACTION OCCURS between your blood and the foods you eat. This reaction is part of your genetic inheritance. It is amazing but true that today, in the twenty-first century, your immune and digestive systems still maintain a memory, a certain favoritism, for foods that your blood type ancestors ate and adapted to.

We know this because of a factor called lectins (from the Latin, "I choose"). Lectins are abundant and diverse proteins found in foods that have agglutinating properties affecting your blood and tissues. Lectins are a powerful way for organisms in nature to attach themselves to other organisms in nature. Lots of germs, and even our own immune systems, use this superglue to their benefit. For example, cells in our liver's bile ducts have lectins on their surfaces to help them snatch up bacteria and parasites. Bacteria and other microbes have lectins on their surfaces as well, which work rather like suction cups, so that they can attach to the slippery mucosal linings of the body. Often the lectins used by viruses or bacteria can be blood type specific, making them a stickier pest for people of that blood type.

So too with the lectins in food. Simply put, when you eat a food containing protein lectins that are incompatible with your blood type antigen, the lectins can attach to the walls of the digestive tract, initiate inflammation, and even penetrate the gut lining and escape into the circulation.

Here's an example of how a lectin agglutinates in the body. Let's say a Type A person eats a plate of lima beans. The lima beans are digested in the stomach through the process of acid hydrolysis. However, the lectin protein is resistant to acid hydrolysis. It doesn't get digested, but stays intact. It may interact directly with the lining of the stomach or intestinal tract, causing inflammation or blocking the absorption of nutrients, or it may even get absorbed into your bloodstream along with the digested lima bean nutrients. Different lectins target different organs and body systems.

Once the intact lectin protein interacts with your tissues, it virtually has a magnetic effect on the cells in that region. It clumps the cells together, which targets them for destruction, as if they too were foreign invaders. This clumping can cause irritable bowel syndrome, disrupt the balance of healthy bacteria in the gut, and even block the absorption of other foods. Some authorities on the subject have even speculated that the lectin-rich diets consumed in third-world and developing countries might be responsible for much of the anemia seen in these populations.

## Lectins: A Dangerous Glue

YOU MAY HAVE HEARD the story of the bizarre assassination of Georgi Markov in 1978 on a London street. Markov was killed while waiting for a bus by an unknown Soviet KGB agent. Initially, the autopsy could not pinpoint how it was done. After a thorough search, a tiny gold bead was discovered embedded in Markov's leg. The bead was found to be permeated with a chemical called ricin, which is a toxic lectin extracted from castor beans. Ricin is so potent an agglutinin that even an infinitesimally small amount can cause death by swiftly converting the body's red blood cells into large clots, which block the arteries. Ricin kills instantaneously. It is so instantly deadly that ricin poisoning has been attempted as a terrorist tool—so far unsuccessfully—and a letter containing ricin is believed to have been sent to President Barack Obama. Ricin also made an appearance on the popular TV series *Breaking Bad*.

Fortunately, most lectins found in the diet are not quite so life threatening, although they can cause a variety of other problems, especially if they are specific to a particular blood type. For the most part, our immune systems protect us from lectins. Ninety-five percent of the lectins we absorb from our typical diets are sloughed off by the body, but at least 5 percent of the lectins we eat are filtered into the bloodstream, where they react with and destroy red and white blood cells. The actions of lectins in the digestive tract can be even more powerful. There they often create a violent inflammation of the sensitive mucus of the intestines, and this agglutinative action may mimic food allergies. Even a minute quantity of a lectin is capable of damaging a huge number of cells if the particular blood type is reactive.

This is not to say that you should suddenly become fearful of every food you eat. After all, lectins are widely abundant in legumes, seafood, grains, and vegetables. It's hard to bypass them. The key is to avoid the lectins that agglutinate your particular cells—determined by blood type. For example, gluten, the most common lectin found in wheat and other grains, binds to the lining of the small intestine, causing substantial inflammation and painful irritation in some blood types—especially Type O.

Lectins vary widely, according to their source. For example, the lectin found in wheat has a different shape from the lectin found in soy, and attaches to a different combination of sugars; each of these foods is dangerous for some blood types, but beneficial for others.

Nervous tissue as a rule is very sensitive to the agglutinating effect of food lectins. This may explain why some researchers feel that allergy-avoidance diets may be of benefit in treating certain types of nervous disorders, such as hyperactivity. Russian researchers have noted that the brains of schizophrenics are more sensitive to the attachment of certain common food lectins. In fact, a Swedish study linked the decline of new schizophrenia cases in Sweden in the years 1940–45 with the lack of bread due to the wartime blockade of wheat shipments. Lectins are also implicated in leptin resistance, a factor in obesity.

Injections of the lentil lectin into the knee joint cavities of nonsensitized rabbits resulted in the development of arthritis that was indistinguishable from rheumatoid arthritis. Many people with arthritis feel that avoiding the nightshade vegetables such as tomatoes, eggplant, and white potatoes seems to help their arthritis. That's not surprising because most nightshades are very high in lectins.

Food lectins can also interact with the surface receptors of the body's white cells, programming them to multiply rapidly. These lectins are called mitogens because they cause the white cells to enter mitosis, the process of cell division. They do not clump blood by gluing cells together; they merely attach themselves to things, like fleas on a dog. Occasionally an emergency room physician will be faced with a very ill but otherwise apparently normal child who has an extraordinarily high white blood cell count. Although pediatric leukemia is usually the first thing to come to mind, the astute physician will ask the parent, "Was your child playing in the yard?" If the answer is yes, "Was he eating any weeds or putting plants in his mouth?" Often it will turn out that the child was eating the leaves or shoots of the pokeweed plant, which contains a lectin with the potent ability to stimulate white cell production.

Finally, if and when lectins penetrate the body's gut defenses and reach the systemic circulation, they can attach to receptors on cells originally designed to receive signals from the body's hormones. Sometimes the lectin can sit on the receptor and block the intended hormone

## Blood Type–Specific Food Lectins

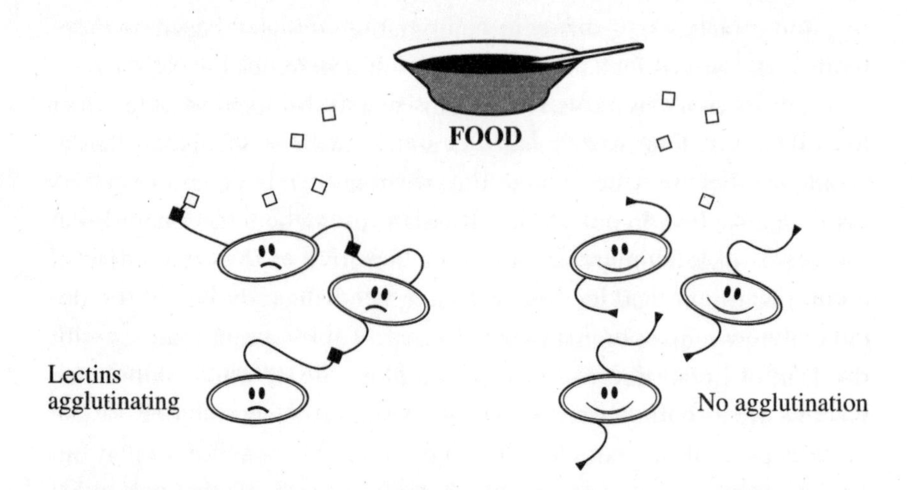


*Each blood type antigen possesses a unique shape; thus, many lectins interact with only one specific blood type because of its form. In the lima bean example, food lectins interact with and agglutinate Type A cells (on the left) because they fit the shape of the A antigen. The antigen for Type B blood (on the right), a different sugar molecule with a different shape, is not affected. Conversely, a food lectin (such as buckwheat) that can specifically attach to and agglutinate cells of Blood Type B would not fit Type A blood.*

from attaching and exerting its effects; other times the lectin can actually stimulate the receptor, making the cell think that the hormone was produced, when in fact it wasn't. From this information, it's possible to conclude that cases of hormonal imbalance could be cured by the simple expedient of intelligent eating.

## Your Personal Ecosystem

Your digestive tract is a hotbed of activity, with a level of interactions rivaling that of a small city. It is estimated that the human digestive tract may contain up to 100 trillion microorganisms, and the human gut may host up to a thousand different species of bacteria. More and more, we hear and read about the importance of the microbiome: the ecological community of friendly and unfriendly microorganisms that share our body space—for both good and ill.

New studies are revealing how the gut microbiome has co-evolved with us and how it manipulates and complements our biology in ways that are mutually beneficial. We are also starting to understand how friendly bacteria operate to improve the integrity and function of the digestive system—and, indeed, the entire human body. For example, consider the microbial profile of an obese person. Obesity appears as the result of a complicated mix of factors such as genetics, environment, diet, and lifestyle, resulting in an imbalance of the equilibrium between energy expenditure and storage in the form of an overabundance of fat. The makeup and interactions of microorganisms and bacteria in the gut are widely recognized as a potential factor in human obesity.

The science of the microbiome is a hot topic in health circles. But clearly not every individual has the same ecosystem. That's where blood type enters the picture. Your blood type antigens are very prominent in your digestive tract. Because of this, many of the bacteria in your digestive tract actually use your blood type molecule as a preferred food supply. Talk about eating right for your blood type! In fact, the blood type's influence is important among intestinal bacteria, almost half of which show some Blood Type A, B, or O specificity.

Simply put, people of different blood types have different gut bacteria. Certain bacteria are 50,000 times more likely to turn up in people with one blood type than another. This originated from our ancestors whose digestive tracts developed to accommodate one type of diet over another, and whose blood types controlled the ability to reject or co-exist with certain bacteria but not others. Our blood type can actually seed our gut by encouraging the growth of only those bacteria strains that can use our blood type antigens as a source of food, while our anti-blood-type antibodies attack bacteria that carry antigens resembling those of a different blood type.

Human feces contain enzymes produced by the bacteria of the microbiome that degrade the ABO blood type antigens lining the digestive tract and convert it to an energy source for their own use. The population of fecal bacteria that produces blood type–degrading enzymes is highly correlated with the blood type of the host. Because many foods have blood type–like antigens, it stands to reason that those foods will be favored by your microbial system.

Harmful lectins in foods can encourage the growth of problematic strains of bacteria, impairing absorption, damaging the intestinal lining, and causing "leaky gut." That is why the first line of support for healing your digestive tract and building a healthy microbiome is eating the right foods for your blood type.

## Secretor Versus Non-Secretor

UP UNTIL NOW we've discussed the role of your blood type antigen as a marker on your cells and tissues. However, in reality there are two forms of the blood type antigen, the one we've been discussing up until this point called the "bound" form that is found in our blood, and another form that floats around in our secretions (tears, digestive juices, perspiration, semen, etc.) called the "unbound" form. Everyone has the ability to make the bound form, where the blood type antigen is attached, and many of us can produce the unbound form as well—but a significant minority are missing the gene for this and cannot. The ability to produce both the bound and unbound form identifies you as a secretor. The inability to produce the unbound form means that you are a non-secretor. Secretors make up about 80 percent of the population; non-secretors, 20 percent.

You might be familiar with the idea of secretor status if you know about law enforcement. For example, a semen sample taken from a rape victim can be used to help convict the rapist if he is a secretor and his blood type matches the blood type identified in the semen. However, if he is in the small population of non-secretors, his blood type cannot be identified from any fluids except the blood because his body does not produce the unbound form of the blood type antigen. (From a practical standpoint, DNA testing makes this less an issue than it once was, although a blood type match is a quick-and-dirty way to know you're on the right track.)

People who do not secrete their blood type antigens in other fluids besides blood are called non-secretors. Being a secretor or a non-secretor

Lower cholesterol
Lower triglycerides
Clearer thinking
Normal blood pressure
Reduced allergy or allergy symptoms
Reduced asthma symptoms
More energy
Better sleep cycle
Chronic pain reduction or resolution
More muscular strength
Fewer seasonal colds and flu
Less bloating and digestive discomfort

4. Take stock of where you're at, using basic measurements: Measure your BMI and waist circumference, along with your weight before you begin (see Chapter Three). If you suffer from a chronic medical condition, it's a good time to record your status, including blood tests.

The Blood Type Diet is not a panacea. But it is a way to restore the natural protective functions of your immune system, reset your metabolic clock, and clear your blood of dangerous agglutinating lectins. It is the best thing you can do to halt the rapid cell deterioration that produces symptoms of aging. And if you have medical problems, this plan can make a critical difference. Depending on the severity of any medical conditions and on the level of compliance with the plan, every person will realize some benefits. That has been my experience, and the experience of my colleagues who use this system with people of all ages and conditions around the world. It makes perfect scientific sense.

In this chapter, I introduce the elements you will find in your Blood Type Diet plan. They are the following:

- The Blood Type Diet
- The Supplement Advisory
- The Stress-Exercise Profile
- The Personality Question

After you read this chapter and review your Blood Type Diet, I suggest you read Part III to get a fuller picture of the specific health and medical implications your plan has for you.

## The Blood Type Diet

YOUR BLOOD TYPE DIET is the restoration of your natural genetic rhythm. The groundwork for the Blood Type Diet was prepared for us many thousands of years ago. Perhaps if we had continued to follow the inherent, instinctual messages of our biological natures, our current condition would be very different. However, human diversity and the sweeping forces of technology intervened.

As we know, because of advantages fighting infections, most early humans were Type O hunters and gatherers who fed on animals, insects, berries, roots, and leaves. The range of dietary choices was extended when humans learned how to raise animals for their own use and how to cultivate crops. But it was not necessarily a smooth and orderly process because not every society adapted well to this change. In many of the early Type O societies, such as the Missouri Valley Indians, the change from a meat-eating diet to an agrarian diet was accompanied by changes in skull formation and the appearance for the first time of dental cavities. Their systems were simply not suited to the newly introduced foods. In other societies, the change from Paleolithic to Neolithic diets appeared to result in shorter statures and less bone density.

Even so, for a long period of time, the traditional agrarian diet provided ample nutrients to avoid malnutrition and support large populations. This changed as advances in agricultural and food processing techniques began to alter foodstuffs even further, increasingly removing them from their natural state. For example, the refining of rice with new milling techniques in twentieth-century Asia caused a scourge of beriberi, a thiamine-deficiency disease, which resulted in millions of deaths.

A more current example is the change from breast-feeding to bottle-feeding in developing countries. The reliance on highly refined, processed infant formula has been responsible for a great deal of malnutrition, diarrhea, and a lowering of the natural immune factors passed on through mother's milk.

Today, it is well accepted that the foods we eat have a direct impact on the state of our health and general well-being. But confusing, and often conflicting, information about nutrition has created a virtual minefield for health-conscious consumers.

How are we to choose which recommendations to follow, and which diet is the right diet? The truth is, we can no more choose the right diet than we can choose our hair color or gender. It was already chosen for us many thousands of years ago.

Without a doubt, much of the confusion is the result of the simplistic one-diet-fits-all premise I spoke of earlier. Although we have seen with our own eyes that certain people respond very well to particular diets while others do not, we have never made a commitment—in science or nutrition—to study the specialized characteristics of populations or individuals that might explain the variety of responses to any given diet. We've been so busy looking at the characteristics of food that we have failed to examine the characteristics of people.

Your Blood Type Diet works because you are able to follow a clear, logical, scientifically based dietary blueprint based on your cellular and genetic profile.

Each of the Blood Type Diets includes twelve food groups:

- Meats and poultry
- Seafood
- Dairy and eggs
- Oils and fats
- Nuts and seeds
- Beans and legumes
- Grains and cereals
- Vegetables
- Fruit
- Beverages, teas and coffee
- Herbs and spices
- Condiments, sweeteners and additives

Each of these groups divides foods into three categories: highly beneficial, neutral, and avoid. Think of the categories this way:

- HIGHLY BENEFICIAL is a food that acts like a medicine. It advances your health or protects you from possible maladies.
- NEUTRAL is a food that acts like a food. It provides required macronutrients and caloric energy.
- AVOID is a food that acts like a poison. It induces biological disorder or increases your chances of disease based on differences between the blood types.

There are a wide variety of foods in each diet, so don't worry about limitations. When possible, show preference for the highly beneficial foods over the neutral foods, but feel free to enjoy the neutral foods that suit you; they won't harm you, and they contain nutrients that are necessary for a balanced diet.

At the top of each food category, you will see a chart that looks like this:

| **BLOOD TYPE O** | | **WEEKLY • IF YOUR ANCESTRY IS** | | |
|---|---|---|---|---|
| *Food* | *Portion* | *African* | *Caucasian* | *Asian* |
| ALL SEAFOOD | 4–6 oz. | 1–4x | 3–5x | 4–6x |

The portion suggestions according to ancestry are not meant as firm rules. My purpose here is to present a way to fine-tune your diet even more, according to what we know about the particulars of your ancestry. Although people of different ethnicities and cultures may share a blood type, there are also geographic and cultural variations. For example, many people of Asian ancestry were not traditionally exposed to dairy products or may not have enough copies of the genes that make the enzyme needed to digest dairy, so they may need to incorporate dairy more slowly into their diets as they adjust their systems to it. The portions are not etched in stone: If you are large-framed and tall, you'll want to steer more to the larger serving and if small-framed and shorter, you'll want the smaller serving. Use the refinements if you think they're helpful; ignore them if you find that they're not. In any case, try to formulate your own plan for portion sizes.

For each Blood Type Diet you'll find three sample menus and several recipes to give you an idea of how you might incorporate the diet into your life. Each blood type has its own reactions to certain foods; these are outlined in your Blood Type Diet. In the first few weeks you'll need to experiment with the guidelines.

The entertainer Liberace was once quoted as saying, "Too much of a good thing is wonderful." However, this may not be true of the Blood Type Diet. I've found that many people assume that the best approach is to religiously eat only highly beneficial foods. While this may be okay for a jump-start, the diet is meant to include a sufficient amount of nutrient-rich neutral foods. The best approach is to eliminate all the foods on your avoid list and reduce those neutral foods for which you can substitute beneficial alternatives. That will leave you with a balanced diet and a healthier method of weight loss.

## The Role of Supplements

YOUR BLOOD TYPE DIET also includes recommendations about vitamin, mineral, and herbal supplements that can enhance the effects of your diet. This is another area in which there is great confusion and misinformation. Popping nutritional supplements is a popular thing to do these days. It's hard not to be seduced by the vast array of remedies overflowing the shelves of your local health food store and advertised online. While there are many ethical manufacturers of dietary supplements, there are others that have no compunction about cutting costs by using low-quality ingredients. A higher-priced formula from a reliable manufacturer may not look as attractive as a lower-priced product you find on the Internet, but be assured there are many hidden factors in that higher cost, such as microbial assays, stability studies, and ingredient standardization. Beware of supplements claiming miracle cures for diseases. Advertising of cures for arthritis and inflammation, heart disease, dementia, cancer, and other serious chronic diseases is not only despicable but also illegal. In my opinion, when used intelligently and with the same degree of personalization as your diet, supplements can have a role in a healthy lifestyle. As with food, nutritional supplements don't always work the same way for everyone. Every vitamin, mineral, and herbal supplement plays a specific role in your body.

You may be unfamiliar with the term *phytochemicals*. Modern science has discovered that many of these phytochemicals, found in plants often called weeds or herbs, are sources of high concentrations of biologically active compounds. Many phytochemicals—which I prefer to think of as food concentrates—are antioxidants, and several of them are many times more powerful than vitamins. It is interesting that, unlike vitamins, phytochemical antioxidants exhibit a remarkable degree of tissue preference. For example, milk thistle (*Silybum marianum*) and the spice turmeric (*Curcuma longa*) both have an antioxidant capability hundreds of times stronger than that of vitamin E, and they have a great degree of preference for liver tissue. These plants are very beneficial for disorders characterized by inflammation of the liver, such as hepatitis and cirrhosis. The health of your gut bacteria will also be enhanced with prebiotics and probiotics, found in food and some supplements—preferably, specific to your blood type.

Your specialized program of vitamins, minerals, and phytochemicals will round out the dietary aspect of your program.

## The Stress-Exercise Connection

IT IS NOT ONLY the foods you eat that determine your well-being. It is also the way your body uses those nutrients for good or ill. That's where stress comes in. The concept of stress is very prominent in modern society. We often hear people remark, "I'm so stressed" or "My problem is too much stress." Indeed, it is true that unbridled stress reactions are associated with many illnesses. Few people realize, though, that it is not the stress itself but our reaction to the stress in our environment that depletes our immune systems and leads to illness. This reaction is as old as human history. It is caused by a natural chemical response to the perception of danger. The best way to describe the stress reaction is to get a mental picture of how the body responds to stress.

Imagine this scenario: You are a man living in a hunting-gathering society. You lie bundled in the dark night, pressed together with your kind, sleeping. Suddenly, a huge animal appears in your midst. Do you grab a weapon and try to fight? Or do you turn and run for your life?

The body's response to stress has been developed and refined over thousands of years. It is a reflex, an animal instinct, our survival mechanism for dealing with life-or-death situations. When danger of any kind is sensed, we mobilize our fight-or-flight response, and we either confront what is alarming us or flee from it—mentally or physically.

Now imagine another scenario: You are in a work cubicle in the offices of a hectic penny stock trading firm. Phones ring constantly, your co-workers are sullen and unsupportive, and more and more work gets dumped into your in-box. Finally, to top it off, you've just seen a memo that several firings will be occurring next week.

The first scenario highlights a type of primordial response to stress. It is produced by a flood of chemicals called catecholamines that cause the adrenal glands to go into overdrive. Your pulse quickens. Your lungs suck in more oxygen to fuel your muscles. Your blood sugar soars to supply a burst of energy. Digestion slows. You break into a sweat. All of these biological responses happen in an instant, triggered by stress. They prepare you—in the same way they prepared our ancient ancestors—for fight or flight. It is a violent biochemical swing in response to an immediate danger. However, like all turbulence, it passes very quickly, which is good, as this type of response is not designed for long-term use.

When the danger passes, your body begins to change again. It starts to calm down and compose itself after the furor caused by the release of so many chemicals. And then, if whatever caused the initial stress is resolved, all of the reactions disappear, and everything is once again copacetic with the body's complex response system. If whatever caused the initial stress continues, the body's ability to adapt to the stress becomes exhausted and the bodily systems eventually shut down.

The second scenario, involving ongoing stress, is quite different.

Unlike the tidal wave of fight-or-flight, this type of stress is low level and ever present. This is the stress of modern living, and it produces a different chemical profile. Unlike the fight-or-flight response of prehistoric humans, which produces a burst of catecholamines, the second type of stress produces a slower chemical response that revolves around the hormone cortisol. This hormone is produced by the adrenal glands according to natural cycles that tend to correlate with the body's internal clock (circadian rhythm). Under stressful situations, cortisol stimulates the production of new glucose from glycogen stores in the liver. Cortisol also blocks the movement of glucose into the cells. All of this means that with high cortisol levels, you will have quite a bit of glucose flying around the bloodstream. A good thing when you are running away from a hungry lion. Not exactly the best thing when you are stressed in everyday life.

Unlike our ancestors, who faced intermittent acute stresses, such as the threat of predators or starvation, we live in a highly pressured, fast-paced world that imposes chronic, prolonged stress. Even though our stress response may be less acute than that of our ancestors, the fact that it is happening continuously may make the consequences even worse. Experts generally agree that the stresses of contemporary society and the resultant diseases—of the body, the mind, and the spirit—are very much a product of our industrialized culture and unnatural style of living.

What is the outcome? Stress-related disorders cause 50 to 80 percent of all illnesses in modern life. We know how powerfully the mind influences the body and the body influences the mind. The entire range of these interactions is still being explored. Problems known to be exacerbated by stress and the mind-body connection are ulcers, high blood pressure, heart disease, migraine headaches, arthritis and other inflammatory diseases, asthma and other respiratory diseases, insomnia and other sleep disorders, anorexia nervosa and other eating disorders, and a variety of skin problems ranging from hives to herpes and from eczema to psoriasis. Stress is disastrous to the immune system, leaving the body open to myriad opportunistic health problems.

Your personal response to stress has a surprisingly strong link to your blood type.

## Catecholamines: Short-Term Stress

Studies have shown that Type O has a stress response that centers on fight-or-flight. The reasons are a bit complicated, so I'll describe it simply here. Dopamine is a major neurotransmitter made by the brain that plays an important role as a chemical messenger and central element in what is called the brain's reward-motivated behavior. Most types of rewards increase the level of dopamine in the brain, and most addictive drugs increase dopamine activity and levels. Dopamine is converted to another neurotransmitter, called norepinephrine (also known as noradrenaline), by an enzyme known as dopamine beta-hydroxylase (DBH).

You can visualize this as two buckets, one high, one low, connected by a tube. The upper bucket is dopamine, the lower bucket norepinephrine, the tube connecting them is DBH. If you're Type O you have a very, very large tube (a lot of DBH), which means that under stress lots of dopamine flows from the upper bucket to the lower one (norepinephrine). Dopamine tends to make us happy and content while norepinephrine tends to make us anxious and prepared for fight-or-flight. A surprising amount of norepinephrine is made in the gut where, in excess, it can disrupt digestion and assimilation and even the balance of the flora.

So under even mild stress, Type O will have to work harder at maintaining dopamine and blunting norepinephrine. Fortunately, there are lifestyle and dietary habits that can accomplish this. For example, vigorous exercise tends to block DBH and narrow the tube a bit, as does a high-protein diet. Wheat, unfortunately, tends to widen the tube, draining dopamine and causing the norepinephrine bucket to overflow.

This higher level of catecholamines can increase feelings of anger and aggression, perhaps explaining why ironically "Type A *behavior*" is in fact associated with Type O blood.

Ever in the middle of things, it is interesting to note that Type Bs appear to have less active DBH (narrower tubes connecting dopamine to norepinephrine) so they tend to have an easier time keeping their dopamine levels up. Perhaps this explains their enviable tendencies toward equanimity.

## Cortisol: Long-Term Stress

It's amazing to see the lengths to which scientists will go to stress out research subjects. In one study designed to measure the levels of cortisol during stress, they made subjects attempt to copy text while looking at their writing in a mirror as they simultaneously listened to a tape loop of a baby crying. When they compared the results by the blood types of the subjects, they made an interesting discovery. Type O (and to a lesser degree Type AB) subjects had a powerful initial spike in their cortisol levels, followed by a rapid drop. Types A and B, on the other hand, had a lower spike, but the elevated levels persisted and persisted.

As we've seen, this prolonged cortisol response is the really dangerous one, and to explain, I'll provide a simple example. Should a person, perhaps due to a motorcycle accident, sustain a traumatic head injury, it is normal procedure in the ER to administer astronomical amounts of corticosteroids in an attempt to reduce the swelling of the brain. Paradoxically, this super-high dose of steroids has virtually no side effects, because it is given over such a short period of time. On the other hand, all of the negative side effects of cortisone medication—immune suppression, weight gain, and cardiovascular disease—take place when you take low doses of cortisone over very long periods of time. The same treatment can heal when administered over a short period and harm when administered over a long time.

That's the same scenario with cortisol. A brief spike is fine, perhaps even desirable. Prolonged elevations cause problems with metabolism, immunity, sleep, and the actions of many, many other genes. This is a real problem for Type As, as they have been shown to have higher incidence of cardiovascular disease and problems associated with lower immunity. If you are Type A and have issues with your metabolism in addition to sleep disturbances, it's likely your cortisol levels are to blame. Fortunately, there are lifestyle habits and dietary changes that can correct this. Perhaps the simplest approach is to begin a program of yoga or tai chi. Both have been shown in reliable studies to reduce cortisol levels.

Many of our internal reactions to stress are ancient tunes being called up and played by our bodies—the environmental stresses that shaped the metabolism of the various blood types. The cataclysmic changes in locale, climate, and diet imprinted these stress patterns into the biochemical memory of each blood type and even today determine our internal response to stress.

Although each of us reacts to stress in a unique way, no one is immune to its effects, especially if it is prolonged and unwanted. Not all stress is bad for you. Certain stresses, such as physical or creative activity, produce pleasant emotional states, which the body perceives as an enjoyably heightened mental or physical experience.

Your Blood Type Diet includes a description of your own blood type stress patterns, along with the recommended course of exercise that will turn stress into a positive force. This element provides a crucial complement to your diet.

## The Personality Question

WITH ALL of these fundamental connections at work, it is not surprising that people might speculate about less tangible characteristics that might be attributed to blood type—such as personality, attitudes, and behavior.

The idea that certain inherited traits, mannerisms, emotional qualities, and life preferences are buried in our genetic makeup is well accepted, although we are only at the very beginning of understanding how this inheritance plays out scientifically. Personality is a mixture of nature and nurture, with nurture probably being the major influence.

Although research has been done linking blood types to personality types, most of it is old, not very good, and subject to the biases common in the time the research was conducted—typically in the 1950s and 1960s. Still, the connection intrigues us because it makes some sense that there might be a causal relationship between what occurs at the cellular level of our beings and our mental, physical, and emotional tendencies as expressed by our blood type. Certainly there must be a link between what we know about the chemical differences between how each blood type responds to stress and at least some elements of personality. For example, higher cortisol levels are associated with obsessive-compulsive disorder (OCD), a condition also known to be more common in Type A. Depression (both unipolar and bipolar) is in part associated with low dopamine levels and has been shown to be more common in Type O.

The belief that personality is determined by one's blood type is held in high regard in Japan. Termed *ketsuekigata*, Japanese blood type analysis is serious business. Corporate managers use it to hire workers, market researchers use it to predict buying habits, and many people use it to choose friends, romantic partners, and lifetime mates. Vending machines that offer on-the-spot blood type analysis are widespread in train stations, department stores, restaurants, and other public places. There is even a highly respected organization, the ABO Society, dedicated to helping individuals and organizations make the right decisions, consistent with blood type.

The leading proponent of the blood type–personality connection is a man named Toshitaka Nomi, whose father first pioneered the theory. In 1980, Nomi and Alexander Besher wrote a book called *You Are Your Blood Type*, which has sold millions of copies in Japan. It contains personality profiles and suggestions for the various blood types—right down to what you should do for a living, whom you should marry, and the dire consequences that might befall you if you should ignore this advice.

It makes for fun reading—not unlike astrology, numerology, or other methods of finding your place in the uncertain scheme of things. I think, however, that most of the advice in the book should be taken with a grain of salt. I don't believe that a soul mate or a romantic partner should be chosen by blood type. I am Type A and I am deeply in love with my wife, Martha, who is Type O. I would hate to think that we might have been kept forever apart because of some psychic incompatibility in our blood types. We do just fine, even though mealtimes can be a little chaotic.

So, what is the value of this speculation, and why am I including it here? It's very simple. Although I think the Japanese *ketsuekigata* is extreme, I can't deny that there is probably an essential truth to the theories about a relationship between differences in physiology and the characteristics of our personalities.

Modern scientists and doctors have clearly acknowledged the existence of a biological mind-body connection, and we've already demonstrated the relationship between your blood type and your response to stress earlier in this chapter. The idea that your blood type may relate to your personality is not really so strange. Indeed, if you look at each of the blood types, you can see a distinct personality emerging—the inheritance of our ancestral strengths. Perhaps this is just another way for you to play to those strengths.

There is as yet not enough hard evidence to justify any sweeping conclusions about the use of blood type to determine personality, but a world of information is waiting to be annexed and explored. For example, a variation in genes known as COMT (catechol *O*-methyltransferase) appears to result in some rather striking differences in personality and appears to even influence whether we can experience the placebo effect. COMT does have some links to the ABO gene, so perhaps history remains to be written in regard to blood types and personality.

It is possible that in this century we will finally be able to examine some master plan, a map that will show us how to get from here to there within ourselves. But perhaps not. There is so much we don't understand, so much we may never understand, but we can speculate, reflect, and consider the many possibilities. That is why we have, as a species, developed such acute intelligence.

These elements—diet, weight management, dietary supplementation, stress control, and personal qualities—form the essential elements of your individual Blood Type Diet. Refer to them often as you begin to familiarize yourself with the specific qualities of your blood type.

But before you go any further, I suggest you do one more thing if you haven't already: Find out your blood type!

PART II

# Your Blood Type Diet

FIVE

# Blood Type

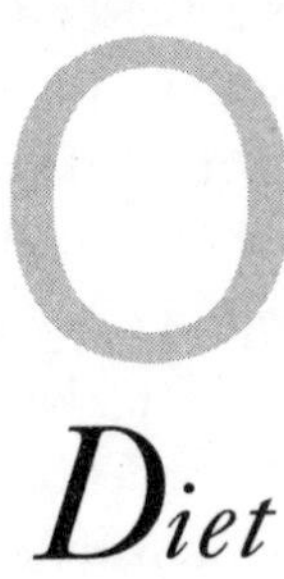

# *Diet*

## TYPE O: *The Hunter*

- Meat eater
- Hardy digestive tract
- Overactive immune system
- Intolerant to dietary and environmental adaptations
- Responds best to stress with intense physical activity
- Requires an efficient metabolism to stay lean and energetic

# The Type O Diet

TYPE O THRIVES on intense physical exercise and animal protein. The digestive tract of Type O retains the memory of ancient times. The high-protein hunter-gatherer diet and the enormous physical demands placed on the system of early Type Os probably kept most primitive humans in a mild state of ketosis—a condition in which the body's metabolism is altered. The body metabolizes proteins and fats into ketones, which are used in place of sugars in an attempt to keep glucose levels steady. The combination of ketosis, calorie deprivation, and constant physical activity made for a lean, mean hunting machine—the key to the survival of the human race.

Dietary recommendations today generally discourage the consumption of too much animal protein because saturated fats have been proven to be a risk factor for heart disease and cancer. Of course, much of the meat consumed today is shot through with fat and tainted by the indiscriminate use of hormones and antibiotics. "You are what you eat" can take on an ominous meaning when you're talking about the modern meat supply. Fortunately, organic and free-range meats are widely available. The success of the Type O diet depends on your use of lean, chemical-free meat and fish along with an abundance of fresh vegetables and fruit.

Type O doesn't find dairy products and grains quite as friendly as do most of the other blood types because its digestive system still has not adapted to them fully. After all, you don't have to chase down and kill a bowl of wheat or a glass of milk! These foods did not become staples of the human diet until much later in the course of our evolution.

NOTE: Longtime readers will notice a difference in the values of a small number of foods between this edition and the original version of *Eat Right for Your Type.* That is because beginning with the publication of *Live Right for Your Type*, I made a distinction in some foods between secretors and non-secretors. The original version of *Eat Right for Your Type*, which preceded *Live Right for*

*Your Type*, "homogenized" these differences. Like all of my subsequent books, this edition of *Eat Right for Your Type* uses the secretor values as the base values for the A, B, AB, and O blood types.

**KEY**

- ‡ Enhances carbohydrate metabolism, helps with weight loss
- ↑ Increases microbiome diversity, discourages microbial imbalance
- ↓ Decreases microbiome diversity, encourages microbial imbalance

## Meats and Poultry

| BLOOD TYPE O | WEEKLY ▪ IF YOUR ANCESTRY IS | | | |
|---|---|---|---|---|
| *Food* | *Portion** | *African* | *Caucasian* | *Asian* |
| LEAN RED MEATS | 4–6 oz. *(men)*<br>2–5 oz. *(women and children)* | 5–7x | 4–6x | 3–5x |
| POULTRY | 4–6 oz. *(men)*<br>2–5 oz. *(women and children)* | 1–2x | 2–3x | 3–4x |

**The portion recommendations are merely guidelines that can help refine your diet according to ancestral propensities.*

Eat lean, chemical- and pesticide-free beef, lamb, beef liver, and venison as a primary protein source. These are your preferred meats, although chicken, turkey, and other neutral poultry products are allowed. The more stressful your job or demanding your exercise program, the higher the grade of protein you should eat. In Type O these are the optimal types of protein for building active tissue mass (calorie-burning tissue) such as muscle, but beware of portion sizes. Try to consume no more than 6 ounces at any one meal (4 to 6 ounces is about the size of the palm of your hand).

Type O can efficiently digest and metabolize meats because it has high stomach acid levels and fat-busting enzymes in abundance. However, Type O must be careful to balance meat proteins with the appropriate vegetables and fruits to provide needed fiber, antioxidants, and micronutrients.

It's very important that Type O choose grass-fed and antibiotic-, hormone-, and pesticide-free meats. These choices are high in conjugated linoleic acid (CLA), a very healthful fatty acid—actually the only trans fat that is good for you. Emphasize eye of round, top round, top sirloin, sirloin tip, brisket, and 95 percent lean ground cuts. These have less of the pro-inflammatory fats.

Optimally, you should look for free-range and grass-fed meats. Grass-fed meat is a natural source of omega-3 fatty acids, whereas grain-fed meat has virtually no omega-3. Be sure poultry is certified organic and is antibiotic- and pesticide-free. Always choose free-range poultry. Select poultry products from the back of the fridge where the temperature is coldest.

Pork naturally contains toxins (biogenic amines) and should be avoided, even organic pork.

### Highly Beneficial

BEEF ↑ ‡
BEEF, HEART ↑
BEEF, LIVER ↑
BEEF, TONGUE
BUFFALO, BISON ↑ ‡
CALF, LIVER ↑
LAMB ↑ ‡
MARROW SOUP
MOOSE ↑
MUTTON ↑ ‡
SWEETBREADS ↑
VEAL ↑ ‡
VENISON ↑

### Neutral

Bear
Bone soup (allowable meats)
Chicken
Chicken liver
Cornish hen
Duck
Goat
Goose

Grouse
Guinea hen
Horse
Ostrich
Partridge
Pheasant
Rabbit
Squab
Squirrel
Turkey

### Avoid

Duck liver
Goose liver
Ham ↓
Pork and bacon ↓
Quail
Turtle

## Seafood

| BLOOD TYPE O | WEEKLY ▪ IF YOUR ANCESTRY IS | | | |
|---|---|---|---|---|
| *Food* | *Portion* | *African* | *Caucasian* | *Asian* |
| ALL SEAFOOD | 4–6 oz. | 1–4x | 3–5x | 4–6x |

Seafood, the second most concentrated animal protein, is well suited for Type O. Seafood can be an excellent protein source. Richly oiled cold-water fish, such as cod and mackerel, are excellent for Type O because they contain the much-needed anti-inflammatory omega-3 fatty acids and help build active tissue (muscle) almost as effectively as red and organ meats. Make sure that your fish is fresh caught, not farm raised, and free of industrial toxins (dioxins, xenobiotics, and heavy metals), which accumulate in the fat. Ask for fish that is nearest to the ice or from the back of the refrigerator where the temperature is coldest.

### Highly Beneficial

BASS, BLUE GILL ↑
BASS, SEA, LAKE ↑
BASS, STRIPED ↑
COD ↑ ‡
HALIBUT ↑ ‡
MACKEREL, SPANISH
PERCH ↑
PERCH, OCEAN ↑
PIKE ↑
RED SNAPPER ↑ ‡
SHAD ↑
SOLE ↑
STURGEON ↑
SWORDFISH ↑
TILEFISH ↑
TROUT, RAINBOW (WILD) ↑ ‡
YELLOWTAIL ↑

## Neutral

Anchovy
Beluga
Bluefish
Bullhead
Butterfish
Carp
Caviar
Chub
Clam
Crab
Croaker
Cusk
Drum
Eel
Flounder
Grouper
Haddock
Hake
Halfmoon fish
Harvest fish
Herring (fresh/pickled/smoked)
Lobster
Mackerel, Atlantic
Mahi-mahi
Monkfish
Mullet
Mussels
Ocean pout
Opaleye fish
Orange roughy
Oyster
Parrotfish
Pickerel, Walleye
Pilchards
Pompano
Porgy
Rosefish
Sailfish
Sailfish roe
Salmon, Atlantic (wild)
Salmon, Chinook
Salmon roe
Salmon, smoked (lox)
Salmon, sockeye
Sardine
Scallop ↑
Scrod
Scup
Sea bream
Shark
Shrimp
Skate
Smelt
Snail, escargot
Sole, gray/Dover
Sucker
Sunfish, pumpkinseed
Tilapia
Trout, sea/steelhead (wild)/brook
Tuna, bluefin/skipjack/yellowfin
Turbot, European
Weakfish
Whitefish
Whiting

## Avoid

Abalone, sea ear, mutton fish ↓
Barracuda
Catfish
Conch
Frog
Muskellunge
Octopus
Pollock, Atlantic
Squid, calamari

## Dairy and Eggs

| BLOOD TYPE O | WEEKLY • IF YOUR ANCESTRY IS | | | |
|---|---|---|---|---|
| *Food* | *Portion* | *African* | *Caucasian* | *Asian* |
| EGGS | 1 EGG | 0 | 4–8X | 5–8X |
| CHEESES | 2 OZ. | 0 | 0–3X | 0–3X |
| MILK | 4–6 OZ. | 0 | 0–1X | 0–2X |

If you're Type O you should severely restrict your consumption of dairy products, a suboptimal protein source for your type. Your system is ill-designed for their proper daily metabolism, and dairy foods can also exacerbate inflammatory conditions and cause weight gain. The sugars commonly encountered in dairy products can also disrupt the Type O microbiome, inhibiting weight loss and leading to digestive problems.

Generally, Type O can eat eggs up to eight times a week. Use eggs from free-range chickens, preferably those advertised as being "DHA rich." DHA is a fatty acid that is increasingly being viewed as essential for proper nerve and immune system health.

### Highly Beneficial

PECORINO CHEESE ↑
ROMANIAN URDA ↑

### Neutral

Butter ↑
Egg white, chicken
Egg whole, chicken
Egg whole, duck
Egg yolk, chicken
Farmer cheese
Feta cheese
Goat cheese
Ghee, clarified butter ↑
Mozzarella cheese, all types

Avoid

American cheese ↓
Blue cheese
Brie cheese
Buttermilk
Camembert cheese ↓
Casein ↓
Cheddar cheese ↓
Colby cheese ↓
Cottage cheese ↓
Cream cheese ↓
Edam cheese ↓
Egg, goose
Egg, quail
Emmental, Swiss cheese ↓
Gorgonzola cheese ↓
Gouda cheese
Gruyère cheese ↓
Half-and-half ↓
Ice cream
Jarlsberg cheese
Kefir ↓
Manchego ↓
Milk, cow (skim or 2% )↓
Milk, cow (whole) ↓
Milk, goat ↓
Monterey Jack cheese ↓
Muenster cheese ↓
Neufchâtel cheese ↓
Paneer cheese ↓
Parmesan cheese
Provolone cheese ↓
Quark cheese ↓
Ricotta cheese ↓
Romano cheese
Roquefort cheese ↓
Sherbet
Sour cream ↓
Stilton cheese ↓
String cheese ↓
Swiss cheese
Whey protein ↓
Yogurt ↓

## Oils and Fats

| BLOOD TYPE O | WEEKLY • IF YOUR ANCESTRY IS | | | |
|---|---|---|---|---|
| *Food* | *Portion* | *African* | *Caucasian* | *Asian* |
| OILS | 1 TABLESPOON | 1–5x | 4–8x | 3–7x |

Type O responds well to many oils. They can be an important source of nutrition and an aid to elimination. You will increase their value in your system if you limit your use to the monounsaturated varieties, such as olive oil and flaxseed oil. These oils have positive effects on the heart and arteries, and may even help reduce blood cholesterol.

Always try to buy high-quality oils, preferably cold pressed when appropriate. Oils do go bad, so make a point of never buying more than you can use within two months.

**Highly Beneficial**

CAMELINA OIL ↑
FLAXSEED, LINSEED OIL ↑ ‡
OLIVE OIL ↑
RICE BRAN OIL

**Neutral**

Almond oil
Apricot kernel oil
Black currant seed oil
Borage seed oil
Canola oil
Chia seed oil
Cod liver oil
Hemp seed oil
Macadamia oil
Perilla seed oil
Pumpkin seed oil
Sesame oil
Walnut oil

**Avoid**

Avocado oil
Castor oil
Coconut oil
Corn oil ↓
Cottonseed oil
Evening primrose oil
Lard
Margarine
Palm oil
Peanut oil
Safflower oil
Soy oil
Sunflower oil
Wheat germ oil

## Nuts and Seeds

| BLOOD TYPE O | WEEKLY • IF YOUR ANCESTRY IS | | | |
|---|---|---|---|---|
| *Food* | *Portion* | *African* | *Caucasian* | *Asian* |
| NUTS AND SEEDS | 6–8 NUTS | 2–5X | 3–4X | 2–3X |
| NUT BUTTERS | 1 TABLESPOON | 3–4X | 3–7X | 2–4X |

Type O can find a good source of supplemental vegetable protein in some varieties of nuts and seeds, while avoiding those with harmful lectins. However, these foods should in no way take the place of high-quality proteins available in meats and seafoods.

Because nuts can sometimes cause digestive problems, be sure to chew them thoroughly or use nut butters, which are easier to digest, especially if you have colon problems, such as diverticulitis.

### Highly Beneficial

CAROB
CHESTNUT, CHINESE ↑
FLAXSEED ↑ ‡
HEMP SEED
PUMPKIN SEED ↑
WALNUT ↑ ‡

### Neutral

Almond ↑
Almond butter ↑
Almond cheese ↑
Almond milk
Butternut
Chia seed
Filbert, hazelnut
Hickory ↑
Macadamia nut
Pecan
Pecan butter↑
Pine nut, pignoli ↑
Safflower seed
Sesame butter, tahini ↑
Sesame flour
Sesame seed ↑
Watermelon seed

### Avoid

Beechnut
Brazil nut
Cashew
Cashew butter
Chestnut, European
Litchi/lychee
Peanut
Peanut butter
Peanut flour
Pistachio nut
Poppy seed
Sunflower butter
Sunflower seed

## Beans and Legumes

| BLOOD TYPE O | WEEKLY • IF YOUR ANCESTRY IS | | | |
|---|---|---|---|---|
| *Food* | *Portion* | *African* | *Caucasian* | *Asian* |
| ALL RECOMMENDED BEANS AND LEGUMES | 1 CUP, DRY | 1–2X | 1–2X | 2–6X |

Type O doesn't utilize beans particularly well. In general, beans inhibit the metabolism of other more important nutrients, such as those found in meat, and a number of them contain lectins that are harmful to Type O. There are a couple of highly beneficial beans that are exceptions and actually strengthen the digestive tract and the balance of the microbiome. Even so, eat beans in moderation, as an occasional side dish.

### Highly Beneficial

ALFALFA SPROUTS
ALOE VERA
ARTICHOKE
BEET GREENS ↑ ‡
BROCCOFLOWER ↑
BROCCOLI ↑ ‡
BROCCOLI RABE, RAPINI ‡
BROCCOLI, CHINESE
CANISTEL ↑
CARROT ↑
CELERY ↑ ‡
CHICORY
COLLARD GREENS ↑ ‡
DANDELION GREENS ‡
ESCAROLE ‡
FENNEL
GARLIC
GINGER
GRAPE LEAVES ↑
HORSERADISH ↑
JERUSALEM ARTICHOKE
KALE ↑
KOHLRABI
LEEK
LETTUCE, ROMAINE
MUSHROOM, MAITAKE, WHITE (COMMON), SILVER DOLLAR ‡
OKRA
ONION, ALL TYPES
PARSLEY
PARSNIP ↑
PUMPKIN ↑ ‡
SEA VEGETABLE, IRISH MOSS
SEA VEGETABLE, KELP, KOMBU, NORI, BLADDERWRACK ↑
SPINACH ↑ ‡
SWISS CHARD ↑ ‡
TOMATILLO ↑
TURNIP
TURNIP GREENS ↑ ‡

### Neutral

Arugula
Asparagus
Asparagus pea
Bamboo shoot
Beet
Bok choy, pak choi
Broccoli leaves
Brussels sprouts
Cassava
Cauliflower
Celeriac
Chayote, pipinella, vegetable pear
Chervil
Chinese kale, Kai-lan
Cilantro
Corn, popcorn
Cucumber
Daikon radish
Endive ↑
Fenugreek ↑
Fiddlehead fern
Hearts of palm
Jicama ↑
Kelp
Lettuce, Bibb, Boston, green leaf, iceberg, mesclun
Mushroom, abalone, black trumpet, enoki, oyster, portobello, straw, tree
Mustard greens ↑
Olive, green
Oyster plant, salsify ↑

Pimiento
Quorn
Radicchio
Radish sprouts
Radish
Rutabaga
Scallion
Sea vegetables, spirulina
Sea vegetables, wakame
Seaweed
Shallot
Squash
Taro leaves, shoots
Water chestnut, matai
Watercress
Zucchini

Avoid

Cabbage ↓
Capers ↓
Eggplant
Juniper
Mushroom, shiitake ↓
Olive, black, Greek, Spanish ↓
Pepper, cayenne, chili, green, jalapeño, red, yellow
Pickles, all
Potato, blue, red, white, yellow ↓
Rhubarb
Sauerkraut ↓
Sweet potato ↓
Tomato
Yam
Yucca

## Fruits

| BLOOD TYPE A | DAILY ▪ ALL ANCESTRAL TYPES | |
|---|---|---|
| *Food* | *Portion* | |
| ALL RECOMMENDED FRUITS | 1 FRUIT OR 3–5 OZ. | 3–4X |

Type A should eat fruits three times a day. Most fruits are allowable, although you should try to emphasize the more alkaline ones, such as berries and plums, which can help balance the grains that are acid forming in your muscle tissues. Melons are also alkaline, but their high mold counts make them hard for Type A to digest. Honeydew melons should be avoided altogether because they have the highest mold counts. Other melons (listed as neutral) can be eaten occasionally.

Type A doesn't do well on tropical fruits, such as mangoes. Although these fruits contain a digestive enzyme that is good for the other blood types, it doesn't work in the Type A digestive tract. Pineapple, on the other hand, is an excellent digestive aid for Type A.

Oranges also should be avoided, as they contain elements that can act like growth factors for undesirable strains of bacteria. This can result in an imbalance of bacteria in the gut, called dysbiosis. Grapefruit, closely related to orange, is an acidic fruit, but it has positive effects on the Type A stomach, exhibiting alkaline tendencies after digestion. Lemons are also excellent for Type A, helping aid digestion and clear mucus from the system.

Because vitamin C is an important antioxidant, especially for stomach cancer prevention, eat vitamin C–rich fruits, such as grapefruit or kiwi.

The banana lectin interferes with Type A digestion. I recommend substituting other high-potassium fruits such as apricots, figs, and allowable melons.

**Highly Beneficial**

APRICOT ↑
BLACKBERRY ‡
BLUEBERRY ‡
BOYSENBERRY
CHERRY ‡
CRANBERRY ↑
FIG ↑
GRAPEFRUIT ↑
JACK FRUIT
LEMON ↑
LIME ↑
PAWPAW
PINEAPPLE ↑ ‡
PLUM ‡
PRUNE ‡

**Neutral**

Acai berry
Apple
Asian pear ↑
Avocado
Breadfruit ↑
Canang melon
Cantaloupe
Casaba melon
Christmas melon
Crenshaw melon
Currant
Date ↑
Dewberry
Durian ↑
Elderberry ↑
Goji, wolfberry
Gooseberry ↑
Grape
Guava ↑
Huckleberry
Kiwi
Kumquat ↑
Lingonberry
Loganberry ↑
Mamey sapote, mamey apple ↑
Mangosteen
Mulberry
Musk melon
Nectarine
Noni
Papaya
Passion fruit ↑
Peach
Pear
Persian melon

Persimmon
Pomegranate
Prickly pear ↑
Quince
Raisin
Raspberry
Sago palm
Spanish melon
Starfruit, carambola
Strawberry
Watermelon
Youngberry

Avoid

Banana
Bitter melon
Coconut
Honeydew melon ↓
Loquat ↓
Mango
Orange ↓
Papaya
Plantain ↓
Tangerine ↓

## Beverages, Teas and Coffee

| BLOOD TYPE A | DAILY ▪ ALL ANCESTRAL TYPES | |
|---|---|---|
| *Food* | *Portion* | |
| ALL RECOMMENDED JUICES | 8 OZ. | 4–5X |
| LEMON AND WATER | 8 OZ. | 1X (IN MORNING) |
| WATER | 8 OZ. | 1–3X |

Type A should start every day with a small glass of warm water into which you have squeezed the juice of half a lemon. This will help reduce the mucus that has accumulated overnight in the more sluggish Type A digestive tract and stimulate normal elimination. Lemon and water also possesses slight, but significant anticlotting effects, helping the Type A's naturally more viscous blood to flow smoother.

Alkaline fruit juices, such as black cherry juice concentrate diluted with water, should be consumed in preference to high-sugar juices, which are more acid forming.

Red wine is good for Type A because of its positive cardiovascular effects. A glass of red wine three or four times a week is believed to lower the risk of heart disease for both men and women.

Coffee may actually be good for Type A. Its antioxidants and enzymes are custom-designed for the Type A digestive tract and immune system. Alternate coffee and green tea for the best combination of benefits.

All other beverages should be avoided. They don't suit the digestive system of Type A, nor do they support the immune system.

Pure fresh water, of course, should be consumed freely.

**Highly Beneficial**

ALFALFA TEA
ALOE JUICE
APRICOT JUICE
BLACKBERRY JUICE
BLUEBERRY JUICE
BURDOCK TEA
CHAMOMILE TEA
CHERRY JUICE
COFFEE ↑
ECHINACEA TEA
FENUGREEK TEA
GINGERROOT TEA
GINSENG TEA
GRAPEFRUIT JUICE ↑
GREEN TEA, KUKICHA, BANCHA, GENMAICHA ↑ ‡
HAWTHORN TEA
LEMON AND WATER ↑
LIME JUICE
MILK, SOY ‡
MILK THISTLE TEA
PINEAPPLE JUICE ↑
PRUNE JUICE
ROSE HIPS TEA
SAINT JOHN'S WORT TEA
SLIPPERY ELM TEA
VALERIAN TEA
VEGETABLE JUICE (FROM HB VEGETABLES)
WINE, RED

**Neutral**

Apple juice, cider
Beet juice
Cabbage juice
Chickweed tea
Coconut water
Coltsfoot tea
Cranberry juice
Cucumber juice
Dandelion tea
Dong quai tea
Elderberry juice
Elder tea
Gentian tea
Goji berry juice
Goldenseal tea
Grape juice
Guava juice
Hops tea
Horehound tea
Licorice root tea
Linden tea
Milk, almond ↑
Milk, rice
Mulberry tea
Mullein tea
Nectarine juice
Noni juice
Parsley tea
Pear juice ↑
Peppermint tea
Pomegranate juice
Raspberry leaf tea

Sage tea
Sarsaparilla tea
Senna tea
Shepherd's purse tea
Skullcap tea
Spearmint tea
Strawberry leaf tea
Thyme tea
Vervain tea
Watermelon juice
White birch tea
White oak bark tea
Wine, white
Yarrow tea
Yerba mate tea

**Avoid**

Beer ↓
Black tea, all forms
Cabbage juice
Catnip tea
Cayenne tea
Coconut milk
Corn silk tea
Liquor, distilled ↓
Mango juice
Orange juice ↓
Papaya juice
Red clover tea
Rhubarb tea
Seltzer water
Soda (such as colas and diet colas)
Tangerine juice ↓
Tomato juice
Yellow dock tea

## Herbs and Spices

Type A should view herbs and spices as more than just flavor enhancers. The right combination of herbs and spices can be powerful immune-system boosters. In fact, spices are the original medicines. Many are rich in anti-microbial essential oils, while others are great sources of anti-oxidants, immune-enhancing phytochemicals and fat-burning thermogenic compounds. Try to include your recommended spices in your diet on a regular basis.

**Highly Beneficial**

DRY MUSTARD
FENNEL
GARLIC
GINGER
HORSERADISH
PARSLEY ↑
TURMERIC

**Neutral**

Allspice
Anise
Arrowroot
Basil
Bay leaf
Bergamot
Caraway
Cardamom
Chervil
Chives
Chocolate
Cilantro
Cinnamon
Clove
Coriander
Cornstarch
Cream of tartar
Cumin
Curry
Dill

Dulse
Guarana
Kelp
Licorice root
Mace
Marjoram
Mustard, dry
Nutmeg
Oregano
Paprika
Peppermint
Rosemary
Saffron
Sage
Salt, sea salt
Savory
Senna
Spearmint
Tarragon
Thyme
Vanilla

**Avoid**

Chili powder
Pepper, black, cayenne, peppercorn, white
Wintergreen

## Condiments, Sweeteners, and Additives

Type A should be careful with condiment use. Blackstrap molasses is a very good source of iron, a mineral that is a bit lacking in the Type A diet. Vinegar should be avoided because the acids tend to cause stomach lining irritation and produce dysbiosis in the gut.

Sugar is allowed in the Type A diet, but only in very small amounts. Use it as you would a condiment, not an energy source. Minimize your use of white processed sugar. Recent studies have shown that the immune system is sluggish for several hours after ingesting it.

**Highly Beneficial**

BARLEY MALT
MISO
MOLASSES
MOLASSES, BLACKSTRAP
SOYBEAN SAUCE, TAMARI, WHEAT FREE

**Neutral**

Agar ↓
Agave syrup ↑
Almond extract
Apple butter
Apple pectin
Baking soda
Brown rice syrup
Carob syrup
Cornstarch
Corn syrup
Dextrose
Fructose
Fruit pectin
Honey
Invert sugar
Jam, jelly (from acceptable fruit)
Lecithin
Maple syrup

Mayonnaise, tofu, soy
Mustard, wheat free, vinegar free ↑
Rice syrup
Salad dressing (low fat from acceptable ingredients)
Stevia
Sugar, brown, white
Umeboshi plum, vinegar
Vegetable glycerine
Yeast, baker's ↑
Yeast, nutritional ↑

### Avoid

Acacia (gum arabic)
Aspartame
Carrageenan ↓
Gelatin ↓
Guar gum
High-fructose corn syrup ↓
High-maltose corn syrup, maltodextrin ↓
Ketchup ↓
MSG
Mayonnaise
Methyl cellulose ↓
Mustard, with vinegar and wheat
Pickle relish ↓
Polysorbate 80 ↓
Sodium carboxy-methyl cellulose ↓
Tamarind
Tragacanth gum ↓
Vinegar, all types ↓
Worcestershire sauce ↓

## Meal Planning for Type A

*Asterisk (*) indicates the recipe is provided.*

THE FOLLOWING sample menus and recipes will give you an idea of a typical diet beneficial to Type A. They were developed by Dina Khader, MS, RD, CDN, a nutritionist who has used the Blood Type Diets successfully with her patients.

These menus are moderate in calories and balanced for metabolic efficiency in Type A. The average person will be able to maintain weight comfortably and even lose weight by following these suggestions. However, alternative food choices are provided if you prefer lighter fare or wish to limit your caloric intake and still eat a balanced, satisfying diet. (The alternative food is listed directly across from the food it replaces.)

Occasionally you will see an ingredient in a recipe that appears on your avoid list. If it is a very small ingredient (such as a dash of pepper), you may be able to tolerate it, depending on your condition and whether you are strictly adhering to the diet. However, the meal selections and recipes are generally designed to work very well for Type As.

As you become more familiar with the Type A diet recommendations, you'll be able to easily create your own menu plans and adjust favorite recipes to make them Type A friendly.

## SAMPLE MEAL PLAN 1

| STANDARD MENU ▪ | WEIGHT-CONTROL ALTERNATIVES ▪ |
|---|---|
| **Breakfast** | |
| water with lemon (on rising) | cornflakes with soy milk and maple syrup or molasses |
| oatmeal with soy milk and maple syrup or molasses | |
| grapefruit juice, coffee, or herbal tea | |
| **Lunch** | |
| Greek salad (chopped lettuce, celery, green onions, cucumber, with a sprinkling of feta cheese, lemon, and fresh mint) | |
| apple | |
| 1 slice sprouted wheat bread | |
| herbal tea | |
| **Midafternoon Snack** | |
| 2 rice cakes with peanut butter | 2 rice cakes with honey |
| 2 plums | |
| green tea or water | |
| **Dinner** | |
| *Tofu-Pesto Lasagna | tofu stir-fry with green beans, leeks, snow peas, and alfalfa sprouts |
| broccoli | |
| frozen yogurt | |
| coffee or herbal tea | |
| (red wine if desired) | |

## SAMPLE MEAL PLAN 2

**Breakfast**

water with lemon (on rising)
*Tofu Omelet
grapefruit juice
coffee or herbal tea

1 poached egg
½ cup low-fat yogurt with sliced berries

**Lunch**

miso soup
mixed green salad
1 slice rye bread
water or herbal tea

**Midafternoon Snack**

*Carob Chip Cookies or yogurt with fruit
herbal tea

*Tofu Dip with raw vegetables

**Dinner**

*Turkey-Tofu Meatballs
steamed zucchini
*String Bean Salad
low-fat frozen yogurt
coffee or herbal tea
(red wine if desired)

## SAMPLE MEAL PLAN 3

**Breakfast**

water with lemon (on rising)
*Maple-Walnut Granola with soy milk
prune, carrot, or vegetable juice
coffee or herbal tea

puffed rice with soy milk

**Lunch**

*Black Bean Soup
mixed green salad

cold salmon on salad greens
with lemon juice and
olive oil

**Midafternoon Snack**

*Apricot Fruit Bread
coffee or herbal tea

½ cup plain yogurt
with drizzle of honey

**Dinner**

*Arabian Baked Fish,
made with bass or whitefish
*Spinach Salad
mixed fresh fruit with yogurt
herbal tea
(red wine if desired)

*Baked Fish

## Recipes

### TOFU-PESTO LASAGNA

*1 pound soft tofu, mashed with*
*2 tablespoons olive oil*
*1 cup shredded part-skim mozzarella cheese or part-skim ricotta*
*1 organic egg (optional)*
*2 packages frozen, chopped spinach or fresh, cut-up spinach*
*1 teaspoon salt*
*1 teaspoon oregano*
*4 cups pesto sauce (you may use less)*
*9 rice or spelt lasagna noodles, cooked*
*1 cup water*

Mix tofu and cheese with egg, spinach, and seasonings. Layer 1 cup sauce in 9 x 13-inch baking dish. Layer noodles, then some of the cheese mixture, then sauce. Repeat, and finish with noodles and sauce on top.
Bake in oven at 350 degrees F. for 30 to 45 minutes or until done.
Makes 4 to 6 servings.

## CAROB CHIP COOKIES

*1/3 cup organic canola oil*
*1/2 cup pure maple syrup*
*1 teaspoon vanilla extract*
*1 organic egg*
*1 3/4 cups oat or brown rice flour*
*1 teaspoon baking soda*
*1/2 cup carob chips (unsweetened)*
*dash allspice (optional)*

Oil two baking sheets and preheat oven to 375 degrees F. In a medium-size mixing bowl, combine the oil, maple syrup, and vanilla. Beat the egg and stir into the oil mixture. Gradually stir in flour and baking soda to form a stiff batter. Fold in carob chips and drop the batter onto the baking sheets by the teaspoon. Bake for 10 to 15 minutes until cookies are lightly browned. Remove from oven and cool.
Makes 3 1/2 to 4 dozen.

## TOFU DIP

*1 cup tofu, mashed*
*1 cup plain nonfat yogurt*
*1 tablespoon olive oil*
*juice of 1 lemon*
*2 tablespoons chopped chives or 1 cup scallions*
*garlic and salt to season*

Combine the tofu, yogurt, olive oil, and lemon juice in a blender and blend at high speed until smooth. Stir in chives or scallions, and

seasonings. Remove to a bowl and refrigerate. If mix is too thick to blend well, add a few drops of water.
Serve dip in a glass bowl centered on a platter of fresh vegetables. Makes approximately 3 cups.

## TOFU OMELET

*1 pound soft tofu, drained and mashed*
*5–6 tree oyster mushrooms, sliced*
*½ pound grated red or white radishes*
*1 teaspoon mirin or sherry for cooking*
*1 teaspoon tamari or soy sauce*
*1 tablespoon fresh parsley*
*1 teaspoon brown rice flour*
*4 organic eggs, lightly beaten*
*1 tablespoon canola or extra-virgin olive oil*

Combine all the ingredients in a mixing bowl, except for oil. Heat the oil in a large frying pan. Pour in half the mixture and cover the pan. Cook over low heat for approximately 15 minutes until egg is cooked. Remove from pan and keep warm.
Repeat the process and use the remainder of the mixture.
Serves 3 to 4.

## TURKEY TOFU MEATBALLS

*1 pound ground turkey*
*1 pound firm tofu*
*½ cup chestnut flour*
*1½ cups spelt flour*
*1 large onion, chopped fine*
*¼ cup fresh parsley, chopped*
*2 teaspoons sea salt*
*4 tablespoons fresh garlic, crushed*
*allowable seasonings to your preference*

Mix well. Refrigerate 1 hour. Roll into small meatballs. To cook, stir-fry in oil until brown and crisp, or bake in the oven at 350 degrees F. for approximately 1 hour.

Makes 4 servings.

---

## STRING BEAN SALAD

*1 pound green string beans*
*juice of 1 lemon*
*3 tablespoons olive oil*
*2 cloves garlic, crushed*
*2 to 3 teaspoons salt*

Wash tender, fresh, green string beans. Remove stems and strings. Cut into 2-inch pieces.

Cook until tender by boiling in plenty of water. Drain. When cool, place in a salad bowl. Dress to taste with lemon juice, olive oil, garlic, and salt.

Makes 4 servings.

---

## MAPLE-WALNUT GRANOLA

*4 cups rolled oats*
*1 cup rice bran*
*1 cup sesame seeds*
*½ cup dried cranberries*
*½ cup dried currants*
*1 cup chopped walnuts*
*1 teaspoon vanilla extract*
*¼ cup organic canola oil*
*¾ cup maple syrup*

Preheat oven to 250 degrees F. In a large mixing bowl combine the oats, rice bran, seeds, dried fruit, nuts, and vanilla. Add the oil and stir evenly.

Pour in maple syrup and mix well until mixture is evenly moistened. Mixture should be crumbly and sticky. Spread mixture on a lightly

oiled cookie tray and bake for 90 minutes, stirring every 15 minutes for even toasting until the mixture is golden brown and dry.
Cool thoroughly and store in airtight container.

---

## BLACK BEAN SOUP

*1 pound black beans*
*2 quarts of water*
*⅛ cup vegetable broth*
*⅛ pound diced white onion*
*⅛ pound green onions plus handful of scallions, for garnish*
*¼ pound celery*
*⅛ pound diced leeks*
*¼ ounce salt*
*1 ounce cumin*
*1 cup dried parsley*
*1 ounce garlic*
*1 medium bunch of fresh tarragon (chopped)*
*1 medium bunch of fresh basil (chopped)*
*1 medium bunch of scallions*

Soak beans in water overnight. Pour off the water and rinse. Add 3 quarts of water and bring beans to a boil.
Discard liquid from the beans and add the vegetable broth. Simmer.
Sauté the onion, celery, leeks, seasonings, and garlic together in a pan. Add this mixture to the beans and continue cooking. Purée ⅛ cup of this soup for consistency. Add scallions at the end for garnish.
Makes approximately 8 servings.

---

## APRICOT FRUIT BREAD

*1¼ cups plain nonfat yogurt*
*1 organic egg*
*1 cup apricot conserves (fruit juice sweetened)*
*2 cups brown rice flour*
*1 teaspoon ground cinnamon*

*1 teaspoon ground allspice*
*1 teaspoon ground nutmeg*
*1¼ teaspoons baking soda*
*1 cup chopped, dried, unsulfured apricots*
*1 cup currants*

Grease a standard-size loaf pan and preheat oven to 350 degrees F. In a medium-size bowl, combine the yogurt, egg, and conserves. Add 1 cup of flour and half of the spices plus baking soda. Stir until batter is evenly moist.

Add remaining flour and spices. If consistency feels too thick, you can add a few drops of cold water or vanilla soy milk to mixture. Fold in apricots and currants.

Pour batter into greased loaf pan and bake for 40 to 45 minutes until done. Remove bread from the pan and cool on a wire rack.

---

## ARABIAN BAKED FISH

*1 large bass or whitefish (3 to 4 pounds)*
*dash of salt to taste*
*¼ cup lemon juice*
*2 tablespoons olive oil*
*2 large onions, chopped and sautéed in olive oil*
*2 to 2½ cups tahini sauce*

Wash fish and dry thoroughly. Sprinkle with salt and lemon juice.

Let stand for 30 minutes. Drain fish. Place in baking pan after brushing with oil. Bake in a preheated oven for 30 minutes at 400 degrees F.

Cover with sautéed onions and tahini sauce, and add a dash of salt. Return to oven and bake until fish is easily flaked with a fork (from 30 to 40 minutes).

Serve the fish on a platter and garnish with parsley and lemon wedges.

Makes 6 to 8 servings.

### TAHINI SAUCE

*1 cup organic tahini*
*juice of 3 lemons*
*2 cloves of garlic, crushed*
*2 to 3 teaspoons salt*
*¼ cup dried, organic parsley flakes or*
*fresh parsley, chopped finely*

In a bowl, mix tahini with lemon juice, garlic, salt, and parsley. Add enough water to make a thick sauce. Makes approximately 2 cups.

---

## BAKED FISH

*1 large whitefish (2 or 3 pounds)*
*or other fish*
*lemon juice*
*salt to taste*
*¼ cup olive oil*
*1 teaspoon cayenne (optional)*
*1 teaspoon pepper (optional)*
*1 teaspoon cumin (optional)*

Wash fish. Sprinkle with salt and lemon juice. Add spices if desired. Let stand for ½ hour. Drain.

Coat fish with oil and place in a baking pan. To prevent fish from drying, wrap with foil, lightly greased with oil. Bake at 350 degrees F. in a preheated oven for 30 to 40 minutes, or until fish is tender and easily flaked.

Makes 4 or 5 servings.

### WITH STUFFING (OPTIONAL)

*⅓ cup pine nuts or shredded almonds*
*2 tablespoons olive oil*
*1 cup parsley, chopped*
*3 cloves garlic, crushed*
*salt, pepper, and allspice to taste*

Sauté nuts in olive oil until lightly browned. Add parsley and spices and sauté for one minute. Stuff raw fish with the mixture.
Makes 4 to 5 servings.

### SPINACH SALAD

*2 bunches fresh spinach*
*1 bunch scallions, chopped*
*juice of 1 lemon*
*¼ tablespoon olive oil*
*salt and pepper to taste (optional)*

Wash spinach well. Drain and chop. Sprinkle with salt. After a few minutes, squeeze excess water. Add scallions, lemon juice, oil, salt and pepper. Serve immediately.
Makes 6 servings.

---

For a wealth of additional recipes in every category, check out the blood type–specific cookbooks and recipe database at dadamo.com and 4yourtype.com.

## Type A Supplement Advisory

THE ROLE OF SUPPLEMENTS—be they vitamins, minerals, or herbs—is to add the nutrients that are lacking in your diet or to provide extra protection where you need it. The supplement focus for Type A is

- Toning the immune system
- Supplying cancer-fighting antioxidants
- Balancing the microbiome
- Strengthening the cardiovascular system

The following recommendations emphasize the supplements that help meet these goals, and warn against the supplements that can be counterproductive or dangerous for Type A.

## Vitamins

### Vitamin $B_{12}$

Type A should be alert to vitamin $B_{12}$ deficiency. Not only is the Type A diet somewhat lacking in this nutrient, which is found mostly in animal proteins, but Type A tends to have a hard time absorbing $B_{12}$ because you lack a substance called "intrinsic factor" in the stomach. (Intrinsic factor is produced by the lining of the stomach and it helps $B_{12}$ be absorbed into the blood.) In elderly Type As, vitamin $B_{12}$ deficiency can cause senile dementia and other neurologic impairments. Look for the methylcobalamin form of the vitamin $B_{12}$ supplement. Avoid the cheaper cyanocobalamin form.

### Other B Vitamins

Most other B vitamins are adequately contained in the Type A diet. If, however, you suffer from anemia, you may want a small supplement of folic acid. Type A heart patients should ask their doctors about low-dose niacin supplements, as niacin has cholesterol-lowering properties.

### Vitamin C

Type A, with higher rates of stomach cancer because of low stomach acid, can benefit from taking additional supplements of vitamin C. Nitrite, a compound that results from the smoking and curing of meats, could be a particular problem for Type A because its cancer-causing potential is greater in people with lower levels of stomach acid. As an antioxidant, vitamin C is known to block this reaction (although you should still avoid smoked and cured foods). However, don't take this to mean that you should take massive amounts. I have found that Type A does not do as well on high doses (1,000 milligrams and up) of vitamin C because it tends to upset the stomach. Taken over the course of a day, two to four capsules of a 250-milligram supplement, preferably derived from rose hips or acerola cherries, should cause no digestive problems.

### Vitamin E

There is some evidence that vitamin E serves as a protectant against both cancer and heart disease—two Type A susceptibilities. You may want to take a daily supplement—no more than 400 IU (International Units).

## Minerals

### CALCIUM

Because the Type A diet includes some dairy products, the need for calcium supplementation is not as acute as for Type O, yet a small amount of additional calcium (300 to 600 milligrams elemental calcium) from middle age onward is advisable. In my experience, Type A does better on particular types of calcium products. The worst source of calcium for Type A is the simplest and most readily available: calcium carbonate (often found in antacids). This form requires the highest amount of stomach acid for absorption. In general, Type As tolerate calcium gluconate, do well on calcium citrate, and do best on a natural calcium derived from the pristine seaweed beds off of northern Ireland, called maerl.

### IRON

The Type A diet is naturally low in iron, which is found in the greatest abundance in red meats. Type A women, especially those with heavy menstrual periods, should be especially careful about keeping sufficient iron stores. If you need iron supplementation, do it under a doctor's supervision, so blood tests can monitor your progress.

In general, use as low a dose as possible, and avoid extended periods of supplementation. Try to avoid crude iron preparations such as ferrous sulfate, which can irritate your stomach. Milder forms of supplementation, such as iron citrate or blackstrap molasses, may be used instead. Floradix, a liquid iron and herb supplement, can be found at most health food stores and is highly assimilable by Type A.

### ZINC

I have found that a small amount of zinc supplementation (as little as 3 milligrams per day) often makes a big difference in protecting children against infections, especially ear infections. Zinc supplementation is a double-edged sword, however. While small, periodic doses enhance immunity, long-term, higher doses depress it and can interfere with the absorption of other minerals. Be careful with zinc!

## Herbs, Phytochemicals, and Probiotics

### Hawthorn

Hawthorn is a great cardiovascular tonic. If you are Type A you should definitely add it to your diet regimen if you or members of your family have a history of heart disease. This phytochemical, with exceptional preventive capacities, is found in the hawthorn tree (*Crataegus oxyacantha*). It has a number of impressive cardiovascular effects. Hawthorn increases the elasticity of the arteries and strengthens the heart, while also lowering blood pressure and exerting a mild solvent-like effect on the plaques in the arteries. Officially approved for pharmaceutical use in Germany, the effects of hawthorn are only now gaining recognition elsewhere. Extracts and tinctures are readily available through naturopathic physicians, health food stores, and pharmacies.

### Immune-Enhancing Herbs

Because the immune system of Type A tends to be open to immune-compromising infections, gentle immune-enhancing herbs, such as purple coneflower (*Echinacea purpurea*), can help ward off colds or flus and may help optimize the immune system's anticancer surveillance. Many people take echinacea in liquid or tablet form. It is widely available. The Chinese herb huang qi (*Astragalus membranaceus*) is also taken as an immune tonic, but is not as easy to find. In both herbs the active ingredients are sugars that act as mitogens that stimulate proliferation of white blood cells, which act in defense of the immune system.

### Chondroitin Sulfate

Chondroitin sulfate is a constituent of our connective tissue and is often sold as a joint-support supplement (along with glucosamine sulfate). Chondroitin is an interesting molecule that turns out to be made up of a long chain of amino sugars that resemble the Blood Type A antigen. In the stomach these chains are broken down and the liberated A-like sugars are free to attract, trap, and block lectins, working more or less as a decoy.

### Calming Herbs

Type A can use mild herbal relaxants, such as chamomile and valerian root, as antistress aids. These herbs are available as teas and should be taken frequently. Valerian has a bit of a pungent odor, which becomes pleasing once you get used to it. There was once a rumor that valerian is so named because it is the natural form of Valium (diazepam), a prescription tranquilizer. This is wrong. Valerian was named for a Roman emperor who had the misfortune to be captured in battle by the Persians. Killed, stuffed, dyed red, and exhibited in a Persian museum, Valerian was fortunate to have had anything named for him. Regardless of the origins of the herb's name, studies show that valerian acts (ever so slightly) on many of the same receptors as do pharmaceutical tranquilizers.

### Quercetin

Quercetin is a bioflavonoid found abundantly in vegetables, particularly yellow onions. Quercetin supplements are widely available, usually in capsules of 100 to 500 milligrams. Quercetin is a very powerful antioxidant, many hundreds of times more potent than vitamin E. It can make a powerful addition to Type A cancer-prevention strategies.

### Milk Thistle

Like quercetin, milk thistle (*Silybum marianum*) is an effective antioxidant with the additional special property of reaching very high concentrations in the liver and bile ducts. Type A can suffer from disorders of the liver and gallbladder. If your family has any history of liver, pancreas, or gallbladder problems, consider adding a milk thistle supplement to your protocol. Cancer patients who are receiving chemotherapy should use a milk thistle supplement to help protect their liver from damage.

### Bromelain (Pineapple Enzymes)

If you are Type A and suffer from bloating or other signs of poor absorption of protein, take a bromelain supplement. This enzyme has a moderate ability to break down dietary proteins, helping the Type A digestive tract assimilate proteins better.

### Probiotic Supplements

If the Type A diet is new for you, you may find that adjusting to a vegetarian diet is uncomfortable and produces excessive gas or bloating. A probiotic supplement can counter this effect by supplying the "good" bacteria usually found in the digestive tract.

## Supplements to Avoid

### Beta-Carotene

My father always avoided giving beta-carotene to his Type A patients, saying that he thought it irritated their blood vessels. I questioned his observation, as it had never been documented. Quite to the contrary, the evidence suggested that beta-carotene could prevent artery disease. Yet recently there have been studies suggesting that beta-carotene in high doses may act as a pro-oxidant, speeding up damage to the tissues rather than stopping it. Perhaps my father's observation was correct, at least in the case of Type A. Vitamin A and beta-carotene can be found in seafood and yellow and orange veggies. This caveat is highly individual: There may be times when a vitamin A supplement is needed for short-term benefits. Check with your doctor.

## Best Carotene-Rich Foods for Type As

| | |
|---|---|
| Egg | Broccoli |
| Spinach | Carrot |
| Yellow squash | |

# Type A Stress-Exercise Profile

The ability to reverse the negative effects of stress lives in your blood type. As we discussed earlier, stress is not in itself a problem; it's how you respond to stress. Each blood type has a distinct, genetically programmed instinct for overcoming stress.

Type A often reacts to stress by mismanaging cortisol, which can cause weight gain, depress the immune system, and interfere with restorative sleep. Even at rest, Type A has higher levels of cortisol than the other blood types. Cortisol-charged bulbs flash in your brain, producing anxiety, irritability, and obsessive tendencies. As the stress signals throb in your immune system, you grow weaker and more tired.

If, however, you adopt a quieting technique, such as yoga or meditation, you can achieve great benefits by countering negative stresses with focus and relaxation. Type A does not respond well to continuous confrontation and needs to consider and practice the art of stillness. If Type A remains in its naturally tense state, stress can produce heart disease and various forms of cancer. Exercises that provide calm and focus are the remedy that pull Type A from the grip of stress.

Tai chi chuan, the slow-motion, ritualistic pattern of Chinese movement, and hatha yoga, the Indian system of yoga commonly practiced in the West, are calming, centering experiences. Moderate isotonic exercises, such as hiking, swimming, and bicycling, are favored for Type As. When I advise calming exercises, it doesn't mean you can't break a sweat. The key is really your mental engagement in your physical activity. For example, heavy competitive sports and exercises will only exhaust your nervous energy, make you tense all over again, and leave your immune system open to illness or disease.

The following exercises are recommended for Type A. Pay special attention to the length of the sessions. To achieve a consistent release of tension and revival of energy, you need to perform one or more of these exercises three or four times a week.

| EXERCISE | DURATION | FREQUENCY (PER WEEK) |
| --- | --- | --- |
| TAI CHI | 30–45 min. | 3–5x |
| HATHA YOGA | 30 min. | 3–5x |
| MARTIAL ARTS | 60 min. | 2–3x |
| GOLF | 60 min. | 2–3x |
| BRISK WALKING | 20–40 min. | 2–3x |
| SWIMMING | 30 min. | 3–4x |
| DANCE | 30–45 min. | 2–3x |

| | | |
|---|---|---|
| AEROBICS (LOW IMPACT) | 30–45 min. | 2–3x |
| STRETCHING | 15 min. | 3–5x |

# Type A Exercise Guidelines

TAI CHI CHUAN, or tai chi, is an exercise that enhances the flexibility of body movement. The slow, graceful, elegant gestures of tai chi routines seem to mask the full-speed hand and foot blows, blocks, and parries they represent. In China, tai chi is practiced daily by groups who gather in public squares to perform the movements in unison. Tai chi can be a very effective relaxation technique, although it takes concentration and patience to master.

Yoga is also good for the Type A stress pattern. It combines inner rectitude with breath control and postures designed to allow for complete concentration without distraction by worldly concerns. If you learn basic yoga postures, you can create a routine best suited to your lifestyle. Many Type As who have adopted yoga relaxation tell me that they will not leave the house until they do their yoga.

## Simple Yoga Relaxation Techniques

Yoga begins and ends with relaxation. We contract our muscles constantly, but rarely do we think of doing the opposite—letting go and relaxing. We can feel better and be healthier if we regularly release the tensions left behind within the muscles by the stresses and strains of life.

The best position for relaxation is lying on your back. Arrange your arms and legs so that you are completely comfortable in your hips, shoulders, and back. The goal of deep relaxation is to let your body and mind settle down to soothing calmness, in the same way that an agitated pool of water eventually calms to stillness.

Begin with abdominal breathing. As a baby breathes, her abdomen moves, not her chest. However, many of us grow to unconsciously adopt the unnatural and inefficient habit of restrained chest breathing. One of the aims of yoga is to make you aware of the true center of breathing. Observe the pattern of your breathing. Is your breathing fast, shallow, and irregular or do you tend to hold your breath? Allow your breathing to revert to a more natural pattern—full, deep, regular, and with no constriction. Try to isolate just your lower breathing muscles; see if you can breathe without moving your chest. Breathing exercises are always done smoothly and without any strain. Place one hand on your navel and feel the movement of your breathing. Relax your shoulders.

Start the exercise by breathing out completely. When you inhale, pretend that a heavy weight, such as a large book, is resting on your navel, and that by your inhalation, you are trying to raise this imaginary weight up toward the ceiling.

Then, when you exhale, simply let this imaginary weight press down against your abdomen, helping you exhale. Exhale more air out than you normally would, as if to "squeeze" more air out of your lungs. This will act as a yoga stretch for the diaphragm and further help release tension in this muscle. Bring your abdominal muscles into play here to assist. When you inhale, direct your breath down so deeply that you are lifting an imaginary heavy weight up toward the ceiling. Try to completely coordinate and isolate the abdominal breath with no chest or rib movement.

Even if you perform aerobic exercises during the course of your week, try to integrate the relaxing, soothing routines that will help you best manage your Type A stress patterns.

SEVEN

# Blood Type B Diet

## TYPE B: *The Nomad*

- Balanced
- Strong immune system
- Tolerant digestive system
- Most flexible dietary choices
- Dairy eater
- Responds best to stress with creativity
- Requires a balance between physical and mental activity to stay lean and sharp

# The Type B Diet

TYPE O AND TYPE A seem to be polar opposites in many respects, but Type B can best be described as idiosyncratic—with utterly unique and sometimes chameleon-like characteristics. In many ways Type B resembles Type O so much that the two seem related. Then, suddenly, Type B will take on a totally unfamiliar shape—one that is peculiarly its own. You might say that Type B represents a sophisticated refinement in the adaptive journey, an effort to join together divergent peoples and cultures.

On the whole, the sturdy and alert Type Bs are usually able to resist many of the most severe diseases common to modern life, such as heart disease and cancer. Even when you do contract these diseases, you are more likely to survive them. Yet because Type Bs are somewhat offbeat, your system seems more prone to exotic neuro-immune system disorders, such as multiple sclerosis, lupus, and chronic fatigue syndrome (see Chapter Eleven).

In my experience, a Type B who carefully follows the recommended diet can often bypass severe disease and live a long and healthy life.

The Type B diet is balanced and wholesome, including a wide variety of foods. In the words of my father, it represents "the best of the animal and vegetable kingdoms." Think of *B* as standing for "balance"—the balancing forces of A and O.

NOTE: Longtime readers will notice a difference in the values of a small number of foods between this edition and the original version of *Eat Right for Your Type.* That is because beginning with the publication of *Live Right for Your Type*, I made a distinction in some foods between secretors and non-secretors. The original version of *Eat Right for Your Type*, which preceded *Live Right for Your Type*, "homogenized" these differences. Like all of my subsequent books, this edition of *Eat Right for Your Type* uses the secretor values as the base values for the A, B, AB, and O blood types.

**KEY**

- ‡ Enhances carbohydrate metabolism, helps with weight loss
- ↑ Increases microbiome diversity, discourages microbial imbalance
- ↓ Decreases microbiome diversity, encourages microbial imbalance

## Meats and Poultry

| BLOOD TYPE B | WEEKLY ▪ IF YOUR ANCESTRY IS | | | |
|---|---|---|---|---|
| *Food* | *Portion** | *African* | *Caucasian* | *Asian* |
| LEAN RED MEATS | 4–6 oz. | 3–4x | 2–3x | 2–3x |
| POULTRY | 4–6 oz. | 0–2x | 0–3x | 0–2x |

**The portion recommendations are merely guidelines that can help refine your diet according to ancestral propensities.*

Type B can derive benefit from selected meats. If you are fatigued or suffer from immune deficiencies, you should eat red meat such as lamb, mutton, or rabbit several times a week, in preference to beef or turkey.

In my experience, one of the most difficult adjustments Type B must make is giving up chicken. Chicken contains a Blood Type B agglutinating lectin in its muscle tissue. If you're accustomed to eating more poultry than red meat, you can eat other poultry such as turkey or pheasant. Although they are similar to chicken in many respects, neither contains the dangerous lectin.

The news about chicken is troubling to many people because it has become a fundamental part of many ethnic diets. In addition, people have been told to eat chicken instead of beef because it is "healthier," but here is another case where one dietary guideline does not fit all.

Chicken may be leaner (although not always) than red meat, but that isn't the issue. The issue is the power of an agglutinating lectin to attack your cells and disrupt your digestion. So, even though chicken may be a beloved food, I urge you to begin weaning yourself from it.

**Highly Beneficial**

GOAT ↑ ‡
LAMB ↑ ‡
MOOSE ↑
MUTTON ↑ ‡
RABBIT ↑
VENISON ↑

**Neutral**

Beef
Beef liver
Beef tongue
Bone soup (allowable meats)
Buffalo, bison
Calf liver
Marrow soup
Ostrich
Pheasant
Turkey
Veal

**Avoid**

Bear
Beef, heart
Chicken ↓
Chicken liver
Cornish hen
Duck
Duck liver
Goose
Goose liver
Grouse
Guinea hen
Ham ↓
Horse
Partridge
Pork and bacon ↓
Quail
Squab
Squirrel
Sweetbreads
Turtle

## Seafood

| BLOOD TYPE B | WEEKLY • IF YOUR ANCESTRY IS | | | |
|---|---|---|---|---|
| *Food* | *Portion* | *African* | *Caucasian* | *Asian* |
| ALL RECOMMENDED SEAFOOD | 4–6 oz. | 4–6x | 3–5x | 3–5x |

### SCRUMPTIOUS FETTUCCINE ALFREDO

*8 ounces rice or spelt fettuccine/linguine*
*1 tablespoon extra-virgin olive oil*
*¾ cup buttermilk*
*⅓ cup plus 2 tablespoons Parmesan cheese (grated)*
*¼ cup sliced scallions*
*2 tablespoons chopped fresh basil or 1 teaspoon dried*
*¼ teaspoon garlic powder or freshly pressed garlic*
*¼ teaspoon finely shredded lemon peel*

Cook pasta according to package directions to the al dente stage.
Drain; immediately return to pan. Add olive oil; toss to coat the pasta.
In same pan as pasta, add buttermilk, ⅓ cup Parmesan cheese, scallions, basil and garlic. Cook everything together over medium-high heat until bubbly, stirring constantly.
Decorate with 2 tablespoons Parmesan cheese and fresh basil.
Serve with lemon.
Makes 4 side dishes.

---

For a wealth of additional recipes in every category, check out the blood type–specific cookbooks and recipe database at dadamo.com and 4yourtype.com.

## Type B Supplement Advisory

The role of supplements—be they vitamins, minerals, or herbs—is to add the nutrients that are lacking in your diet and to provide extra protection where you need it. The supplement focus for Type B is

- Fine-tuning an already balanced diet
- Improving metabolic efficiency
- Strengthening immunity
- Improving brain clarity and focus

Type B is a special (you might say lucky) case. For the most part, you can avoid major diseases by following your Blood Type Diet. Because your diet is so rich in vitamin A, vitamin B, vitamin E, vitamin C, calcium, and iron, there is no need for supplementation of these vitamins and minerals. So enjoy your unique status—but follow your diet!

The following are the few supplements that can benefit Type B individuals.

## Minerals

### MAGNESIUM

While the other blood types risk calcium deficiency, Type B risks magnesium deficiency. Magnesium is the catalyst for the metabolic machinery in Type B. It's the match head—what makes Type B metabolize carbohydrates more efficiently. Because you are so efficient in assimilating calcium, you risk creating an imbalance between your levels of calcium and magnesium. Should this occur, you find yourself more at risk for viruses (or otherwise lowered immunity), fatigue, depression, and, potentially, nervous disorders. In these instances, perhaps a trial of magnesium supplementation (300 to 500 milligrams) should be considered. Also, many Type B children are plagued with eczema, and magnesium supplementation can often be beneficial. Any form of magnesium is fine, although more patients report a laxative effect with magnesium citrate than with the other forms. An excessive amount of magnesium could, at least theoretically, upset your body's calcium levels, so be sure that you consume high-calcium foods as well, such as cultured dairy products. The key is balance!

## Herbs, Phytochemicals, and Probiotics

### LICORICE

Licorice (*Glycyrrhiza glabra*) is a plant widely used by herbalists around the world. It has at least four uses: as a treatment for stomach ulcers, as an antiviral agent against the herpes virus, to treat chronic fatigue syndrome, and to combat hypoglycemia. Licorice is a plant to be respected; large doses in the wrong person can cause sodium retention and elevated blood pressure. If you are Type B and suffer from hypoglycemia, a condition in which the blood sugar drops after a meal, drink a cup or two of licorice tea after meals. If you suffer from chronic fatigue syndrome, I recommend that you use licorice preparations, other than deglycyrrhizinated licorice (DGL) and licorice tea, only under the guidance of a physician. Licorice freely used in its supplemental form can be toxic.

### Modified Citrus Pectin

Modified citrus pectin (MCP) is a special type of pectin, a molecule found in many, if not most, plants. Pectin is widely used in cooking as a thickener. MCP (and pectin in general) is composed of a long chain of a sugar that bears striking resemblance to the Type B antigen. In the stomach, the acids break the chains up, liberating the sugar, which can then act to attract, block, and defuse Type B–specific lectins. This has been extensively studied in regard to blocking lectins from attaching to the tissues of the liver. MCP can be found in some health food stores, from naturopathic physicians, and online.

### Digestive Enzymes

If you are a Type B who is not used to eating meat or dairy foods, you may experience some initial difficulties adapting to your diet. Take a digestive enzyme with your main meals for a while, and you'll adjust more readily to concentrated proteins. Bromelain, an enzyme found in pineapples, is available in supplemental form.

### Adaptogenic Herbs

Adaptogenic herbs increase concentration and memory retention, sometimes a problem for Type Bs who have nervous or viral disorders. The best are Siberian ginseng (*Eleutherococcus senticosus*) and ginkgo biloba, both widely available. Siberian ginseng has been shown in Russian studies to increase the speed and accuracy of teletype operators. Ginkgo biloba is currently the most frequently prescribed drug of any kind in Germany, where more than 5 million people take it daily. Ginkgo increases the microcirculation to the brain, which is why it is often prescribed to the elderly.

LECITHIN. Lecithin, a blood enhancer found principally in soy, allows the cell-surface B antigens to move around more easily and better protect the immune system. Type B should seek this benefit from lecithin granules, not soy itself, as soy doesn't have the concentrated effect. Drinking the Membrosia Cocktail is a good habit to develop, as it allows you to get an excellent modulator for your nervous and immune systems in a rather pleasant way.

## Type B Stress-Exercise Profile

TYPE B responds to stress in ways that tend to resemble that of Type A and destresses in ways that resemble Type O. Type B shares the tendency for higher cortisol levels with Type A, but because their levels of the dopamine-busting enzyme DBH are on the low side, they somewhat compensate for this.

As a Type B, you confront stress very well for the most part because you blend more easily into unfamiliar situations. You're less anxious or aggressive than Type O and less physically impacted than Type A. Thus Type B does well with exercises that are neither too aerobically intense nor completely aimed at mental relaxation. The ideal balance for many Type Bs consists of moderate activities that involve other people—such as group hiking, biking excursions, the less aggressive martial arts, tennis, and aerobics classes. You don't do as well when the sport is fiercely competitive—such as squash, football, or basketball.

The most effective exercise schedule for Type B should be three days a week of more intense physical activity and two days a week of relaxation exercises.

| EXERCISE | DURATION | FREQUENCY (PER WEEK) |
| --- | --- | --- |
| AEROBICS | 45–60 min. | 3x |
| TENNIS | 45–60 min. | 3x |
| MARTIAL ARTS | 30–60 min. | 3x |

| | | |
|---|---|---|
| CALISTHENICS | 30–45 min. | 3x |
| HIKING | 30–60 min. | 3x |
| CYCLING | 45–60 min. | 3x |
| SWIMMING | 30–45 min. | 3x |
| BRISK WALKING | 30–60 min. | 3x |
| JOGGING | 30–45 min. | 3x |
| WEIGHT TRAINING | 30–45 min. | 3x |
| GOLF | 60 min. | 2x |
| TAI CHI | 45 min. | 2x |
| HATHA YOGA | 45 min. | 2x |

# Type B Exercise Guidelines

The three components of a high-intensity exercise program are the warm-up period, the aerobic exercise period, and a cool-down period. A warm-up is very important to prevent injuries, because it brings blood to the muscles, readying them for exercise, whether it is walking, running, biking, swimming, or playing a sport. A warm-up should include stretching and flexibility movements to prevent muscle and tendon tears.

The exercises can be divided into two basic types: isometric exercises, in which stress is created against stationary muscles, and isotonic exercises, such as calisthenics, running, or swimming, which produce muscular resistance through a range of movement. Isometric exercises can be used to tone up specific muscles, which can then be further strengthened by isotonic exercise. Isometrics may be performed by pushing or pulling an immovable object or by contracting or tightening opposing muscles.

To achieve maximum cardiovascular benefits from aerobic exercise, you must elevate your heart rate to approximately 70 percent of your maximum. Once that elevated rate is achieved during exercise, continue exercising to maintain that rate for 30 minutes. This regimen should be repeated at least three times each week.

To calculate your maximum heart rate:

1. Subtract your age from 220.
2. Multiply the difference by 70 percent (.70). If you are over sixty years of age, or in poor physical condition, multiply the remainder by 60 percent (.60).
3. Multiply the remainder by 50 percent (.50). For example, a healthy fifty-year-old woman would subtract 50 from 220, for a maximum heart rate of 170. Multiplying 170 by .70 would give her 119 beats per minute, which is the top level she should strive for. Multiplying 170 by .50 would give her the lowest number in her range.

### FOR RELAXATION EXERCISES

Tai chi and yoga are the perfect way to balance the more physical activities of your week.

Tai chi chuan, or tai chi, is an exercise that enhances the flexibility of body movement. The slow, graceful, elegant gestures of tai chi seem to mask the full-speed hand and foot blows, blocks, and parries they represent. In China, tai chi is practiced daily by groups who gather in public squares to perform the movements in unison. Tai chi can be a very effective relaxation technique, although it takes concentration and patience to master.

Yoga combines inner rectitude with breath control and postures designed to allow for complete concentration without distraction by worldly concerns. Hatha yoga is the most common form of yoga practiced in the West. If you learn basic yoga postures, you can create a routine best suited to your lifestyle.

Some patients have told me that they are concerned that adopting yoga practices may conflict with their religious beliefs. They fear that the practice of yoga implies that they have adopted Eastern mysticism. I respond, "If you eat Italian food, does that make you Italian?" Meditation and yoga are what you make of them. Visualize and meditate on the subjects that are relevant to you. The postures are neutral; they are just timeless and proven movements.

## SIMPLE YOGA RELAXATION TECHNIQUES

Yoga begins and ends with relaxation. We contract our muscles constantly, but rarely do we think of doing the opposite—letting go and relaxing. We can feel better and be healthier if we regularly release the tensions left behind within the muscles by the stresses and strains of life.

The best position for relaxation is lying on your back. Arrange your arms and legs so that you are completely comfortable in your hips, shoulders, and back. The goal of deep relaxation is to let your body and mind settle down to soothing calmness, in the same way that an agitated pool of water eventually calms to stillness.

Begin with abdominal breathing. As a baby breathes, her abdomen moves, not her chest. However, many of us grow to unconsciously adopt the unnatural and inefficient habit of restrained chest breathing. One of the aims of yoga is to make you aware of the true center of breathing. Observe the pattern of your breathing. Is your breathing fast, shallow, and irregular or do you tend to hold your breath? Allow your breathing to revert to a more natural pattern—full, deep, regular, and with no constriction. Try to isolate just your lower breathing muscles; see if you can breathe without moving your chest. Breathing exercises are always done smoothly and without any strain. Place one hand on your navel and feel the movement of your breathing. Relax your shoulders.

Start the exercise by breathing out completely. When you inhale, pretend that a heavy weight, such as a large book, is resting on your navel, and that by your inhalation, you are trying to raise this imaginary weight up toward the ceiling.

Then, when you exhale, simply let this imaginary weight press down against your abdomen, helping you exhale. Exhale more air out than you normally would, as if to "squeeze" more air out of your lungs. This will act as a yoga stretch for the diaphragm and further help release tension in this muscle. Bring your abdominal muscles into play here to assist. When you inhale, direct your breath down so deeply that you are lifting an imaginary heavy weight up toward the ceiling. Try to completely coordinate and isolate the abdominal breath with no chest or rib movement.

EIGHT

# Blood Type AB Diet

## TYPE AB: *The Enigma*

- Modern merging of A and B
- Chameleon's response to changing environmental and dietary conditions
- Sensitive digestive tract
- Overly tolerant immune system
- Responds best to stress spiritually, with physical verve and creative energy
- An evolutionary mystery

# The Type AB Diet

BLOOD TYPE AB is rare (2 to 5 percent of the population), and biologically complex. It doesn't fit comfortably into any of the other categories. Multiple antigens make Type AB sometimes A-like, sometimes B-like, and sometimes a fusion of both—kind of a blood type centaur.

This multiplicity of qualities can be positive or negative, depending on the circumstances, so the Type AB diet requires that you read your foods lists very carefully and familiarize yourself with both the Type A and Type B diets to better understand the parameters of your own diet.

Essentially, most foods contraindicated for either Type A or Type B are probably bad for Type AB—although there are some exceptions. Panhemagglutinins, which are lectins capable of agglutinating all of the blood types, seem to be better tolerated by Type AB, perhaps because the lectin reaction is diminished by the double A and B antibodies. Tomatoes are an excellent example. Type A and Type B cannot tolerate the lectins, while Type AB eats tomatoes with no discernible effect.

Type AB is often stronger and more active than the more sedentary Type A. This extra dollop of élan vital may be because Type AB's genetic memory still contains fairly recent remnants of its steppe-dwelling Type B ancestors.

NOTE: Longtime readers will notice a difference in the values of a small number of foods between this edition and the original version of *Eat Right for Your Type.* That is because beginning with the publication of *Live Right for Your Type,* I made a distinction in some foods between secretors and non-secretors. The original version of *Eat Right for Your Type,* which preceded *Live Right for Your Type,* "homogenized" these differences. Like all of my subsequent books, this edition of *Eat Right for Your Type* uses the secretor values as the base values for the A, B, AB, and O blood types.

**KEY**

- ‡ Enhances carbohydrate metabolism, helps with weight loss
- ↑ Increases microbiome diversity, discourages microbial imbalance
- ↓ Decreases microbiome diversity, encourages microbial imbalance

## Meats and Poultry

| BLOOD TYPE AB | WEEKLY ▪ IF YOUR ANCESTRY IS | | | |
|---|---|---|---|---|
| *Food* | *Portion** | *African* | *Caucasian* | *Asian* |
| LEAN RED MEATS | 4–6 oz. | 1–3x | 1–3x | 1–3x |
| POULTRY | 4–6 oz. (men) | 0–2x | 0–2x | 0–2x |

**The portion recommendations are merely guidelines that can help refine your diet according to ancestral propensities.*

When it comes to eating meat and poultry, Type AB borrows characteristics from both Type A and Type B. Like Type A, you do not produce enough stomach acid to effectively digest too much animal protein. Yet the key is portion size and frequency. Type AB needs some meat protein, especially the kinds that play to its B-like traits—lamb, mutton, rabbit, and turkey, instead of beef. The lectin in chicken that irritates the blood vessels and digestive tracts of Type B has the same effect on Type AB, so stay away from chicken.

Also avoid all smoked or cured meats. These foods can cause stomach cancer in people with low levels of stomach acid, the trait you share with Type A.

**Highly Beneficial**

TURKEY ↑ ‡

**Neutral**

Beef liver
Calf liver
Goat
Lamb
Mutton
Ostrich
Pheasant
Rabbit

**Avoid**

Bear
Beef
Beef heart
Beef tongue
Bone soup
(allowable meats)
Buffalo, bison
Caribou
Chicken ↓
Chicken liver
Cornish hen
Duck
Duck liver
Goose
Goose liver
Grouse
Guinea hen
Horse
Kangaroo
Marrow soup
Moose
Opossum
Partridge
Pork and bacon ↓
Quail
Squab
Squirrel
Sweetbreads
Turtle
Veal
Venison

## Seafood

| BLOOD TYPE AB | WEEKLY ▪ IF YOUR ANCESTRY IS | | | |
|---|---|---|---|---|
| *Food* | *Portion* | *African* | *Caucasian* | *Asian* |
| ALL RECOMMENDED SEAFOOD | 4–6 oz. | 3–5x | 3–5x | 4–6x |

There is a wide variety of seafoods for Type AB, and it is an excellent source of protein for you. Like Type A, your digestive tract may experience problems from the lectins found in some whitefish, such as sole and flounder. The edible snail, *Helix aspersa/pomatia* (escargot), contains a powerful lectin that may help prevent some cancers that Type AB individuals appear more prone to developing.

**Highly Beneficial**

COD ↑ ‡
GROUPER ↑
MACKEREL, ATLANTIC ↑ ‡
MAHI-MAHI ↑
MONKFISH ↑
PICKEREL, WALLEYE ↑
PIKE ↑
PORGY ↑
RED SNAPPER ↑
SAILFISH
SAILFISH ROE
SALMON, ATLANTIC (WILD) ↑
SALMON, CHINOOK ↑
SALMON, SOCKEYE ↑
SARDINE ↑
SHAD ↑ ‡
SNAIL, ESCARGOT ↑
STURGEON ↑
TUNA, BLUEFIN ↑
TUNA, SKIPJACK
TUNA, YELLOWFIN

**Neutral**

Abalone, sea ear, mutton fish
Bluefish
Bullhead
Butterfish
Carp
Catfish
Caviar
Chub
Croaker
Cusk
Drum
Halfmoon fish
Harvest fish
Herring
Mackerel, Spanish
Mullet
Muskellunge
Mussel
Ocean pout
Opaleye fish
Orange roughy
Parrotfish
Perch
Perch, ocean
Pilchards
Pollock, Atlantic
Pompano
Rosefish
Scallop
Scrod
Scup
Sea bream
Shark
Smelt
Squid, calamari
Sucker
Sunfish, pumpkinseed
Swordfish
Tilapia
Tilefish
Weakfish
Whitefish

**Avoid**

Anchovy
Barracuda
Bass, blue gill
Bass, sea, lake
Bass, striped ↓
Beluga
Clam
Conch
Crab

Crayfish
Eel ↓
Flounder
Frog
Haddock
Hake
Halibut
Herring, pickled, smoked
Lobster
Lox (smoked salmon)
Octopus
Oyster ↓
Salmon roe
Shrimp
Skate
Sole
Trout, rainbow (wild)
Trout, sea
Trout, steelhead (wild)
Whiting
Yellowfish
Yellowtail

## Dairy and Eggs

| BLOOD TYPE AB | WEEKLY • IF YOUR ANCESTRY IS | | | |
|---|---|---|---|---|
| *Food* | *Portion* | *African* | *Caucasian* | *Asian* |
| EGGS | 1 EGG | 3–5x | 3–4x | 2–3x |
| CHEESES | 2 OZ. | 2–3x | 3–4x | 3–4x |
| YOGURT | 4–6 OZ. | 2–3x | 3–4x | 1–3x |
| MILK | 4–6 OZ. | 1–6x | 3–6x | 2–5x |

For dairy foods, Type AB can put on the "B" hat, benefiting from dairy foods, especially cultured and soured products—yogurt, kefir, and nonfat sour cream—which are more easily digested and help develop a healthy microbiome.

The primary factor you have to watch out for is excessive mucus production. Like Type A, you already produce a lot of mucus, and you don't need more. Watch for signs of respiratory problems, sinus attacks, or ear infections, which might indicate you should cut back on the dairy foods.

Eggs are a very good source of protein for Type AB. Although they're high in cholesterol and Type AB (like Type A) has some susceptibility to heart conditions, research has shown that the biggest culprits in elevated cholesterol are not cholesterol-containing foods but rather saturated fats.

**Highly Beneficial**

COTTAGE CHEESE ↑
EGG WHITE, CHICKEN ↑
FARMER CHEESE
FETA CHEESE
GOAT CHEESE
KEFIR ↑
MANCHEGO CHEESE
MILK, GOAT ‡
MOZZARELLA CHEESE, ALL TYPES
PECORINO CHEESE ↑
RICOTTA CHEESE
ROMANIAN URDA ↑
SOUR CREAM ↑
YOGURT

**Neutral**

Casein
Caviar
Cheddar cheese
Colby cheese
Cream cheese
Edam cheese
Egg, goose
Egg, quail
Egg whole, chicken
Egg yolk, chicken
Emmental, Swiss cheese
Ghee, clarified butter ↑
Gouda cheese ↑
Gruyère cheese
Jarlsberg cheese ↑
Milk, cow (skim or 2%)
Monterey Jack cheese
Muenster cheese
Neufchâtel cheese
Paneer cheese
Quark cheese
Stilton cheese
String cheese
Swiss cheese
Whey protein

**Avoid**

American cheese ↓
Blue cheese
Brie cheese
Butter
Buttermilk
Camembert cheese ↓
Egg, duck
Gorgonzola cheese ↓
Half-and-half ↓
Ice cream
Milk, cow (whole)
Parmesan cheese
Provolone cheese ↓
Romano cheese
Roquefort cheese ↓
Sherbet

## Oils and Fats

| BLOOD TYPE AB | WEEKLY ▪ IF YOUR ANCESTRY IS | | | |
|---|---|---|---|---|
| *Food* | *Portion* | *African* | *Caucasian* | *Asian* |
| OILS | 1 TABLESPOON | 1–5x | 4–8x | 3–7x |

Type AB should use olive oil rather than animal fats, hydrogenated vegetable fats, or other vegetable oils. Olive oil is a monounsaturated fat that is believed to contribute to lower blood cholesterol. You may also use small amounts of ghee, a semifluid clarified butter popular in India, in your cooking. Walnut oil, which can be added to salads, can help promote cell cleansing, especially in the brain and nervous system, a process called autophagy.

### Highly Beneficial

APRICOT KERNEL OIL
CAMELINA OIL ↑
HEMP SEED OIL
OLIVE OIL ↑ ‡
WALNUT OIL ↑ ‡

### Neutral

Almond oil
Black currant seed oil
Borage seed oil
Canola oil
Castor oil
Chia seed oil
Cod liver oil
Evening primrose oil
Flaxseed, linseed oil
Hazelnut oil
Macadamia oil
Peanut oil
Perilla seed oil
Rice bran oil
Soybean oil
Wheat germ oil

### Avoid

Avocado oil
Coconut oil
Corn oil ↓
Cottonseed oil
Lard
Margarine
Palm oil
Pumpkin seed oil
Safflower oil ↓
Sesame oil ↓
Sunflower oil ↓

## Nuts and Seeds

| BLOOD TYPE AB | WEEKLY • IF YOUR ANCESTRY IS | | | |
|---|---|---|---|---|
| *Food* | *Portion* | *African* | *Caucasian* | *Asian* |
| NUTS AND SEEDS | 6–8 NUTS | 2–5X | 2–5X | 2–3X |
| NUT BUTTERS | 1 TABLESPOON | 3–7X | 3–7X | 2–4X |

Nuts and seeds present an unclear picture for Type AB individuals. Choose carefully, eat them in small amounts and consume with caution. Although they can be a good supplementary protein source, seeds are a common source of food lectins, and your double AB antigens afford them ample opportunities for mischief.

### Highly Beneficial

CHESTNUT, CHINESE ↑
CHESTNUT, EUROPEAN ↑
PEANUT ↑ ‡
PEANUT BUTTER ↑
PEANUT FLOUR ↑
WALNUT ↑ ‡

### Neutral

Almond ↑
Almond butter ↑
Almond cheese ↑
Almond milk
Beechnut
Brazil nut ↑
Butternut ↑
Carob ↑
Cashew ↑
Cashew butter
Chia seed ↑
Flaxseed ↑
Hemp seed ↑
Hickory ↑
Litchi/lychee
Macadamia ↑
Pecan ↑
Pecan butter
Pine nut, pignoli ↑
Pistachio ↑
Safflower seed
Watermelon seed

### Avoid

Filbert, hazelnut
Poppy seed
Pumpkin seed
Sesame butter, tahini

Sesame flour
Sesame seed
Sunflower butter
Sunflower seed

## Beans and Legumes

| BLOOD TYPE AB | WEEKLY ▪ IF YOUR ANCESTRY IS | | | |
|---|---|---|---|---|
| *Food* | *Portion* | *African* | *Caucasian* | *Asian* |
| ALL BEANS AND LEGUMES | 1 CUP, DRY | 3–5X | 2–3X | 4–6X |

Beans and legumes are another mixed bag for Type AB. Like seeds, beans are a rich source of food lectins, and like seeds, your double antigen setup gives them twice the opportunity for mayhem. Some of these foods are idiosyncratic to Type AB.

Like Type A, Type AB should make soybean products, like tofu, a regular part of their diet in combination with small amounts of meat and dairy.

### Highly Beneficial

LENTIL, GREEN
NATTO ↑
NAVY BEANS
PINTO BEANS
PINTO BEANS, SPROUTED ↑
SOYBEAN
SOYBEAN CHEESE
SOYBEAN, SPROUTED ↑
SOYBEAN, TEMPEH ↑
SOYBEAN, TOFU ‡
SOY, MISO

### Neutral

Cannellini beans
Copper beans
Great Northern beans ↑
Green beans
Jicama
Lentils, sprouted
Lentils, all types
Peas
Snap beans
Soybean granules, lecithin
Soybean meal
Soybean pasta ↑
Soy cheese
Soy milk
String beans
Tamarind beans ↑
White beans

**Avoid**

Adzuki beans
Black beans
Black-eyed peas ↓
Broad beans, fava ↓
Butter beans ↓
Garbanzo beans, chickpeas ↓
Haricot-vert
Kidney beans ↓
Lima beans ↓
Lima bean flour ↓
Mung beans, sprouts ↓

## Grains and Cereals

| BLOOD TYPE AB | DAILY ▪ IF YOUR ANCESTRY IS | | | |
|---|---|---|---|---|
| *Food* | *Portion* | *African* | *Caucasian* | *Asian* |
| BREADS, CRACKERS | 1 SLICE | 0–1X | 0–1X | 0–1X |
| MUFFINS | 1 MUFFIN | 0–1X | 0–1X | 0–1X |
| GRAINS | 1 CUP, DRY | 2–3X | 3–4X | 3–4X |
| PASTA | 1 CUP, DRY | 2–3X | 3–4X | 3–4X |

Guidelines for Type AB favor both Type A and Type B recommendations. Generally, you do well on grains, even wheat, but need to limit your wheat consumption. Wheat is also not advised if you are trying to lose weight. Type ABs with a pronounced mucus condition, caused by asthma or frequent infections, should also limit wheat consumption.

Limit your intake of wheat germ and bran to once a week. Oatmeal, soy flakes, millet, and soy granules are good Type AB cereals, but you must avoid buckwheat and corn.

Be aware that sprouted wheat breads sold commercially often contain small amounts of sprouted wheat and are basically whole wheat breads. Look for 100 percent sprouted breads (usually called Manna or Essene bread). Read the ingredient labels.

If you're Type AB, you'll benefit from a diet that includes more rice than pasta, although you may have semolina or spinach pasta once or twice a week. Again, avoid corn and buckwheat in favor of oats and rye.

### Highly Beneficial

AMARANTH
ESSENE, MANNA BREAD
FONIO
JOB'S TEARS, (*COIX* SPP.)
MALANGA, TANNIA, *XANTHOSOMA* ↑
MILLET
OAT BRAN
OATMEAL, OAT FLOUR, OATS
RICE BRAN
RICE FLOUR, BROWN
RICE, BASMATI
RICE, BROWN
RICE, PUFFED, CAKES
RICE, WHITE
RICE, WILD
RYE
RYE BERRY
RYE FLOUR
SOYBEAN FLOUR ‡
SPELT, WHOLE GRAIN

### Neutral

Barley ↑
Black bean flour
Cream of rice
Emmer
Flaxseed bread (containing allowable grains) ↑
Graham flour
Larch fiber
Lentil flour, dahl
Mastic gum
Papadum
Puffed wheat
Quinoa ↑
Rice flour, white
Shredded wheat
Spelt flour, noodles
Taro, Tahitian, poi, dasheen
Wheat, bran, germ
Wheat, bulgur
Wheat, durum, semolina, couscous
Wheat, whole grain flour, white flour

### Avoid

Artichoke flour, pasta ↓
Buckwheat, kasha, soba ↓
Cornflakes
Cornmeal, hominy, polenta ↓
Garbanzo bean (chickpea) flour
Grits
Kamut
Lima bean flour
Sorghum
Tapioca, manioc, cassava, yucca ↓
Teff

## Vegetables

| BLOOD TYPE AB | DAILY • ALL ANCESTRAL TYPES | |
|---|---|---|
| *Food* | *Portion* | |
| RAW VEGETABLES | 1 CUP, PREPARED | 3–5x |
| COOKED OR STEAMED | 1 CUP, PREPARED | 3–5x |

Fresh vegetables are an important source of phytochemicals, the natural substances in foods that have a tonic effect in cancer and heart disease prevention. They should be eaten several times a day. Type AB has a wide selection—nearly all the vegetables that are good for either Type A or Type B are good for you as well.

The one interesting exception is the panhemagglutinin in tomatoes, which affects all blood types. Since Type AB has so much blood type material and the lectin isn't specific, you seem able to avoid the ill effects.

Like Type B, you must avoid fresh corn and all corn-based products.

### Highly Beneficial

ALFALFA SPROUTS
BEET
BEET GREENS ↑ ‡
BROCCOFLOWER ↑
BROCCOLI ↑ ‡
BROCCOLI, CHINESE
CANISTEL ↑
CAULIFLOWER ‡
CELERY ↑ ‡
COLLARD GREENS ↑ ‡
CUCUMBER ↑ ‡
DANDELION GREENS
EGGPLANT ↑ ‡
GARLIC
GRAPE LEAVES ↑
HEART OF PALM ↑
KALE ↑
MUSHROOMS, MAITAKE ‡
MUSTARD GREENS ↑ ‡
PARSLEY
PARSNIP ↑
SEA VEGETABLES, IRISH MOSS
SEA VEGETABLES, SPIRULINA
SWEET POTATO
TURNIP GREENS ↑ ‡
YAM

**Neutral**

Arugula
Asparagus
Asparagus peas
Bamboo shoot
Bok choy, pak choi
Broccoli leaves
Broccoli rabe, rapini
Brussels sprouts
Cabbage
Carrots
Celeriac
Chayote, pipinella, vegetable pear
Chervil
Chicory
Chinese kale, Kai-lan
Cilantro
Daikon radish
Endive ↑
Escarole
Fennel
Fiddlehead fern
Ginger ↑
Horseradish ↑
Jicama ↑
Kohlrabi ↑
Leeks
Lettuce, green leaf, Bibb, Boston, iceberg, mesclun, romaine
Mushroom, black trumpet
Mushroom, enoki
Mushroom, oyster
Mushroom, portobello
Mushroom, straw
Mushroom, white, silver dollar
Okra
Olive, green
Onion, all types
Oyster plant, salsify ↑
Pepper, bell
Pimiento
Potato, blue, red, yellow, white with skin
Pumpkin
Quorn
Radicchio
Rutabaga
Sauerkraut
Scallion
Sea vegetables, kelp, kombu, nori, bladderwrack ↑
Sea vegetables, wakame
Shallot
Spinach
Squash
Swiss chard
Taro leaves, shoots
Tomatillo
Tomato
Turnip
Water chestnut, matai
Watercress
Zucchini

**Avoid**

Aloe vera ↓
Artichoke ↓
Avocado ↓
Capers ↓
Cassava ↓
Corn, popcorn ↓
Fenugreek ↓
Jerusalem artichoke ↓
Mushroom, shiitake ↓
Olive, black ↓
Pepper, chili, jalapeño
Pickles, all
Radish
Radish, sprouted
Rhubarb

## Fruits

| BLOOD TYPE AB | DAILY ▪ ALL ANCESTRAL TYPES | |
|---|---|---|
| *Food* | *Portion* | |
| ALL RECOMMENDED FRUITS | 1 FRUIT OR 3–5 OZ. | 3–4X |

Type AB inherits mostly Type A intolerances and preferences for certain fruits. Emphasize the more alkaline fruits, such as grapes, plums, and berries, which can help balance the grains that are acid forming in your muscle tissues.

Type AB doesn't do particularly well on certain tropical fruits—in particular mangoes and guava—but pineapple is an excellent digestive aid for Type AB.

Oranges also should be avoided, as they can undo some of the good gut rehabilitation that occurs with the diet. Grapefruit is closely related to oranges and is also an acidic fruit, but it has positive effects on the Type AB stomach, exhibiting alkaline tendencies after digestion. Lemons also are excellent for Type AB, aiding digestion and clearing mucus from the system.

Because vitamin C is an important antioxidant, especially for stomach cancer prevention, eat other vitamin C–rich fruits, such as grapefruit or kiwi.

The banana lectin interferes with Type AB digestion. I recommend substituting other high-potassium fruits such as apricots, figs, and certain melons.

### Highly Beneficial

CHERRY ‡
CRANBERRY ↑ ‡
FIG ↑
GOOSEBERRY ‡
GRAPEFRUIT ↑
GRAPE ↑
JACK FRUIT
KIWI ↑
LEMON ↑
LOGANBERRY ‡
MAMEY SAPOTE, MAMEY APPLE ↑
PAWPAW
PINEAPPLE ↑ ‡
PLUM
WATERMELON

### Neutral

Acai berry
Apple
Apricot
Asian pear ↑
Blackberry
Blueberry
Boysenberry↑
Breadfruit ↑
Canang melon
Cantaloupe
Casaba
Christmas melon
Crenshaw melon
Currant
Date ↑
Durian ↑
Elderberry ↑
Goji, wolfberry
Honeydew
Kumquat ↑
Lime
Lingonberry
Mangosteen
Mulberry
Musk melon
Nectarine
Noni
Papaya
Passion fruit ↑
Peach
Pear
Persian melon
Plantain
Prune
Raisin
Raspberry
Spanish melon
Strawberry
Tangerine
Youngberry

### Avoid

Avocado
Banana
Bitter melon
Coconut
Dewberry
Guava
Huckleberry
Loquat ↓
Mango
Orange ↓
Persimmon ↓
Pomegranate ↓
Prickly pear
Quince
Sago palm
Starfruit, carambola

## Beverages, Teas and Coffee

| BLOOD TYPE AB | DAILY ▪ ALL ANCESTRAL TYPES | |
|---|---|---|
| *Food* | *Portion* | |
| ALL RECOMMENDED JUICES | 8 oz. | 2–3x |
| WATER | 8 oz. | 4–7x |

Type AB individuals should begin each day by drinking a glass of warm water with the freshly squeezed juice of half a lemon to cleanse the system of mucus accumulated while sleeping. It also has a very mild blood-thinning effect that is desirable for Type AB and aids elimination. Follow with a diluted glass of grapefruit or papaya juice. In general, choose high-alkaline fruit juices such as black cherry, cranberry, or grape.

A glass of red wine three or four times a week can be beneficial for Type AB because of its positive cardiovascular effects. Replace coffee with green tea for the greatest benefit. Green tea has powerful antioxidant qualities, important for Type AB individuals.

### Highly Beneficial

ALFALFA TEA
BURDOCK TEA
CHAMOMILE TEA
CHERRY JUICE
CRANBERRY JUICE ↑
ECHINACEA TEA
GINSENG TEA
GRAPE JUICE
GREEN TEA, KUKICHA, BANCHA, GENMAICHA ↑ ‡
HAWTHORN TEA
LEMON AND WATER ↑
MILK, RICE
PINEAPPLE JUICE ↑
ROSE HIPS TEA
STRAWBERRY LEAF TEA
VEGETABLE JUICE (FROM HB VEGETABLES)
WATERMELON JUICE

### Neutral

Apple cider, juice
Apricot juice
Beer
Blackberry juice
Blueberry juice
Catnip tea
Cayenne tea
Chickweed tea
Cucumber juice
Club soda
Dandelion tea
Dong quai tea
Elderberry juice
Elder tea
Gingerroot tea
Goldenseal tea
Grapefruit juice
Horehound tea
Licorice root tea
Milk, almond ↑
Milk, soy
Mulberry tea
Nectarine juice
Noni juice
Papaya
Parsley tea
Pear juice ↑
Peppermint tea
Prune juice
Raspberry leaf tea
Sage tea
Saint John's wort tea
Sarsaparilla tea
Seltzer water
Slippery elm tea
Spearmint tea

Tangerine juice
Thyme tea
Tomato juice
Valerian tea
Vervain tea
White birch tea
White oak bark tea
Wine, red
Wine, white
Yarrow tea
Yellow dock tea
Yerba mate tea

**Avoid**

Aloe tea
Black tea, all forms
Coconut milk
Coffee
Coltsfoot tea
Corn silk tea
Fenugreek tea
Gentian tea
Guava juice
Hops tea
Linden tea
Liquor, distilled ↓
Mango juice
Mullein tea
Orange juice ↓
Pomegranate juice
Red clover tea
Rhubarb tea
Senna tea
Shepherd's purse tea
Skullcap tea
Soda, cola, diet cola, misc.

## Herbs and Spices

Spices were the original medicine, so think of them that way. Many herbs and spices are rich in antimicrobial essential oils, while others are great sources of antioxidants, immune-enhancing phytochemicals, and fat-burning thermogenic compounds. Try to work your recommended spices into your diet on a regular basis.

Avoid all pepper and vinegar because they tend to unbalance the absorption machinery of the digestive tract. Instead of vinegar, use lemon juice with oil and herbs to dress vegetables or salads.

And don't be afraid to use generous amounts of garlic. It's a potent tonic and natural antibiotic, especially for Type AB.

Sugar and chocolate are allowed in small amounts. Use them as you would condiments.

**Highly Beneficial**

CURRY
GARLIC
GINGER
HORSERADISH
OREGANO ↑
PARSLEY ↑

### Neutral

- Arrowroot
- Basil
- Bay leaf
- Bergamot
- Caraway
- Cardamom
- Chervil
- Chili powder
- Chive
- Chocolate
- Cilantro
- Cinnamon
- Clove
- Coriander
- Cream of tartar
- Cumin
- Dill
- Dulse
- Fennel
- Ginger ↑
- Kelp
- Licorice root
- Mace
- Marjoram
- Mustard, dry
- Nutmeg
- Paprika
- Peppermint
- Rosemary
- Saffron
- Sage
- Salt, sea salt
- Savory
- Senna
- Spearmint
- Tarragon
- Thyme
- Turmeric
- Vanilla
- Wintergreen

### Avoid

- Allspice
- Anise
- Guarana
- Pepper, black ↓
- Pepper, red flakes ↓

## Condiments, Sweeteners and Additives

Be sure to avoid all pickled condiments, due to their negative effect on the microbiome. Also avoid ketchup, which contains vinegar.

### Highly Beneficial

MISO ‡
MOLASSES, BLACKSTRAP

### Neutral

- Agar
- Agave syrup ↑
- Apple butter
- Apple pectin
- Baking soda
- Brown rice syrup
- Carob syrup
- Fructose
- Fruit pectin
- Honey
- Jams, jelly (with acceptable fruits)
- Lecithin
- Maple syrup
- Mayonnaise
- Mayonnaise, tofu, soy
- Molasses
- Mustard, wheat free, vinegar free ↑
- Rice syrup
- Salad dressing from acceptable ingredients

Soybean sauce, tamari, wheat free
Stevia
Sugar, brown, white
Umeboshi plum, vinegar
Vegetable glycerine
Yeast, baker's ↑
Yeast, brewer's ↑

Avoid

Acacia (gum arabic)
Aloe
Almond extract
Aspartame
Barley malt ↓
Carob syrup
Carrageenan ↓
Cornstarch ↓
Dextrose ↓
Gelatin
Guar gum
High-fructose corn syrup ↓
High-maltose corn syrup, maltodextrin ↓
Invert sugar
Ketchup ↓
Methyl cellulose ↓
MSG
Mustard, with vinegar and wheat
Pickle relish ↓
Polysorbate 80 ↓
Sodium carboxymethyl cellulose ↓
Soy sauce
Sucanat
Tragacanth gum ↓
Vinegar, all types ↓
Worcestershire sauce ↓

## Meal Planning for Type AB

*Asterisk (*) indicates the recipe is provided.*

THE FOLLOWING SAMPLE menus and recipes will give you an idea of a typical diet beneficial to Type ABs. They were developed by Dina Khader, MS, RD, CDN, a nutritionist who has used the Blood Type Diet successfully with her patients.

These menus are moderate in calories and balanced for metabolic efficiency in Type AB. The average person will be able to comfortably maintain weight and even lose weight by following these suggestions. However, alternative food choices are provided if you prefer lighter fare or wish to limit your caloric intake and still eat a balanced, satisfying diet. (The alternative food is listed directly across from the food it replaces.)

Occasionally you will see an ingredient in a recipe that appears on your avoid list. If it is a very small ingredient (such as a dash of pepper), you may be able to tolerate it, depending on your condition and whether you are strictly adhering to the diet. However, the meal selections and recipes are generally designed to work very well for Type ABs.

As you become more familiar with the Type AB diet recommendations, you'll be able to easily create your own menu plans and adjust favorite recipes to make them Type AB–friendly.

| STANDARD MENU ▪ | WEIGHT-CONTROL ALTERNATIVES ▪ |
|---|---|

## SAMPLE MEAL PLAN 1

| **Breakfast** | |
|---|---|
| water with lemon (on rising) | |
| 8 ounces diluted grapefruit juice | |
| 2 slices Essene bread | 1 slice Essene bread |
| *Yogurt-Herb Cheese | 1 poached egg |
| coffee | |
| **Lunch** | |
| 4 ounces sliced turkey breast | |
| 2 slices rye bread | 1 slice rye bread or 2 rye crisps |
| Caesar salad | |
| 2 plums | |
| herbal tea | |
| **Midafternoon Snack** | |
| *Tofu Cheesecake | ½ cup low-fat yogurt with fruit |
| iced herbal tea | |
| **Dinner** | |
| *Tofu Omelet | |
| stir-fried vegetables | |
| mixed fruit salad | |
| decaffeinated coffee | |
| (red wine if desired) | |

## SAMPLE MEAL PLAN 2

**Breakfast**
water with lemon (on rising)
diluted grapefruit juice
*Maple-Walnut Granola with soy milk
coffee

**Lunch**
*Tabbouleh
bunch of grapes or apple
iced herbal tea

**Midafternoon Snack**
*Carob Chip Cookies
coffee or herbal tea

honeydew melon with a scoop of cottage cheese

**Dinner**
*Baked Rabbit
*String Bean Salad
basmati rice
frozen yogurt
decaffeinated coffee
(red wine if desired)

steamed broccoli and cauliflower

## SAMPLE MEAL PLAN 3

**Breakfast**
water with lemon (on rising)
diluted grapefruit juice
1 poached egg
2 slices Essene bread with organic almond butter
coffee

1 slice Essene bread with low-sugar jam

**Lunch**
*Tofu-Sardine Fritters
or
*Tofu-Pesto Lasagna
mixed green salad
2 plums
herbal tea

tofu-vegetable stir-fry

**Midafternoon Snack**
fruit juice–sweetened yogurt

**Dinner**
broiled salmon with fresh dill and lemon
*Saffron Brown Rice
*Spinach Salad
decaffeinated coffee
(red wine if desired)

asparagus

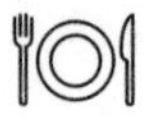

# Recipes

## YOGURT-HERB CHEESE

*2 32-ounce containers of plain nonfat yogurt*
*2 cloves minced garlic*
*1 teaspoon thyme*
*1 teaspoon basil*
*1 teaspoon oregano*
*salt and pepper to taste*
*1 tablespoon olive oil*

Spoon yogurt into an old pillowcase or cheesecloth. Tie the cheesecloth with string and allow the yogurt to drip over a kitchen sink or a bathtub for 4½ to 5 hours.

Remove yogurt from cheesecloth and mix it with all the spices and oil in a bowl. Cover and chill for 1 to 2 hours before serving. Great served with raw vegetables.

---

## TOFU CHEESECAKE (BAKED) (RECIPE BY YVONNE CHAPMAN)

*1½ pounds pressed tofu*
*⅔ cup soy milk*
*¼ teaspoon salt (optional)*
*2 teaspoons fresh lemon juice*
*grated rind of one lemon*
*1 teaspoon vanilla extract*

Blend all ingredients together.

### PIE CRUST

*¾ cup whole meal flour (or rye flour)*
*½ cup oatmeal*
*½ teaspoon salt*
*½ cup oil*
*2 tablespoons cold water*

Combine ingredients, stir in oil, then water, until mixture holds together. Press over bottom and sides of an 8-inch pie pan. Prick bottom several times with a fork. Fill pie crust with tofu mixture and bake at 300 degrees F. for 30 to 45 minutes.

Makes approximately 8 servings.

## TOFU OMELET

*1 pound soft tofu, drained and mashed*
*5–6 portobello mushrooms, sliced*
*½ pound grated scallions*
*1 teaspoon mirin or sherry for cooking*
*1 teaspoon wheat-free tamari or soy sauce*
*1 tablespoon fresh parsley, chopped*
*1 teaspoon brown rice flour*
*4 organic eggs, lightly beaten*
*choice of allowable seasonings to taste*
*2 teaspoons organic extra-virgin olive oil*

Combine all the ingredients except for oil. Heat the oil in a large frying pan. Pour in half the mixture and cover the pan. Cook over low heat for approximately 15 minutes until egg is cooked. Remove from pan and keep warm.

Repeat the process and use the remainder of the mixture.

Serves 3 to 4.

## MAPLE-WALNUT GRANOLA

*4 cups rolled oats*
*1 cup rice bran*
*½ cup dried currants*
*½ cup dried cranberries*
*1 cup minced walnuts or almonds*
*1 teaspoon vanilla extract*
*¼ cup organic canola oil*
*¾ cup maple syrup*

Preheat oven to 250 degrees F. In a large mixing bowl combine the oats, rice bran, dried fruit, nuts, and vanilla. Add the oil and stir evenly.

Pour in maple syrup and mix well until evenly moistened. Mixture should be crumbly and sticky. Spread mixture in a cookie tray and bake for 90 minutes, stirring every 15 minutes for even toasting until the mixture is golden brown and dry.

Cool well and store in airtight container.

---

## TABBOULEH

*1 cup millet, cooked*
*1 bunch green onions, chopped*
*4 bunches parsley, chopped*
*1 bunch mint, chopped, or 2 tablespoons dried mint*
*1 large cucumber, peeled and chopped (optional)*
*⅓ cup olive oil*
*juice of 3 lemons*
*1 tablespoon salt*

Place millet in a large bowl. Add all chopped vegetables and mix well. Add oil, lemon juice, and salt. Serve over fresh green lettuce. Eat with lettuce leaves, tender grape leaves, or with a fork. Makes a refreshing appetizer or a picnic salad.

Makes 4 servings.

---

## CAROB CHIP COOKIES

*⅓ cup organic canola oil*
*½ cup pure maple syrup*
*1 teaspoon vanilla extract*
*1 organic egg*
*1 teaspoon baking soda*
*1¾ cups oat or brown rice flour*
*½ cup carob chips (unsweetened)*

Oil two baking sheets and preheat oven to 375 degrees F. In a medium-size mixing bowl, combine the oil, maple syrup and vanilla. Beat the egg and stir into the oil mixture. Gradually stir in soda and flour to form a stiff batter. Fold in carob chips and drop the batter onto

the baking sheets by the teaspoon. Bake for 10 to 15 minutes until cookie is lightly browned. Remove from oven and cool.
Makes 3½ to 4 dozen.

---

## GRILLED RABBIT

*2 rabbits*
*1 cup apple cider vinegar*
*1 small onion, chopped*
*2 teaspoons salt*
*¼ cup water*
*1 cup rice flour or crushed wheat-free bread crumbs*
*¼ teaspoon pepper*
*dash of cinnamon*
*⅓ cup margarine*

Clean dressed rabbits and cut into serving pieces. Marinate meat in vinegar, onion, and salted water for a few hours before cooking. Drain.
Combine flour, salt and spices in a plate. Dip pieces in melted margarine, then in flour or crushed bread crumb mixture until well coated.
Grill in oven at 375 degrees F. for 30 to 40 minutes.
Makes 4 to 6 servings.

---

## STRING BEAN SALAD

*1 pound green string beans*
*juice of 1 lemon*
*3 tablespoons olive oil*
*2 cloves garlic, crushed*
*2 to 3 teaspoons salt*

Wash tender, fresh, green string beans. Remove stems and strings. Cut into 2-inch pieces.
Cook until tender by boiling in plenty of water. Drain. When cool, place in a salad bowl. Dress to taste with lemon juice, olive oil, garlic, and salt.
Makes 4 servings.

## TOFU SARDINE FRITTERS (RECIPE BY YVONNE CHAPMAN)

*1 can deboned sardines*
*2 1-inch slices of medium or firm tofu*
*¼ teaspoon horseradish powder*
*dash of cider vinegar*
*olive oil*

Mash sardines with a fork until fluffy. Mash tofu into the sardines.

Sprinkle in the horseradish powder. Add a dash of vinegar. Continue mixing ingredients until well blended.

Form into small patties. Heat a small amount of olive oil in a heavy skillet. Brown both sides of patties, or alternatively brown on a grill. This recipe goes well with a salad.

Serves 2.

## TOFU-PESTO LASAGNA

*1 pound soft tofu, mashed with 2 tablespoons olive oil*
*1 cup shredded mozzarella cheese (part skim) or part-skim ricotta*
*1 organic egg (optional)*
*2 packages frozen, chopped spinach or fresh, cut-up spinach*
*1 cup water*
*1 teaspoon salt*
*1 teaspoon oregano*
*9 rice or spelt lasagna noodles, cooked*
*4 cups pesto sauce (you may use less)*

Mix tofu and cheese with egg, spinach, water, and seasonings.

Layer 1 cup sauce in 9 x 13 baking dish. Layer noodles, then cheese mixture, and then sauce. Repeat and end with noodles and sauce on top. Bake in oven at 350 degrees F. for 30 to 45 minutes or until done.

## SAFFRON BROWN RICE

*3 tablespoons extra-virgin olive oil*
*1 large Spanish onion or red onion*
*1 teaspoon ground coriander*
*1 teaspoon nutmeg*
*2 cardamom pods (use only seeds from inside)*
*1 teaspoon saffron threads*
*2 tablespoons rose water (found in Middle Eastern stores)*
*2 cups brown basmati rice*
*4 cups filtered water (boiling)*

Heat the oil and sauté onion with all spices for 10 minutes on low heat. In a separate dish beat the saffron and add to rose water in a small bowl.

To the onion mixture, add 1 tablespoon rose water. Simmer for another 15 minutes and then add the rice with boiling water. Cook for 35 to 40 minutes. Just before serving add the rest of the rose water.

Makes 4 servings.

## SPINACH SALAD

*2 packages fresh spinach*
*1 bunch scallions, chopped*
*juice of 1 lemon*
*¼ tablespoon olive oil or flaxseed oil*
*salt and pepper to taste*
*hot pepper (optional)*

Wash spinach well. Drain and chop. Sprinkle with salt. After a few minutes, squeeze excess water. Add scallions, lemon juice, oil, salt and pepper. Serve immediately.

Makes 6 servings.

---

For a wealth of additional recipes in every category, check out the blood type–specific cookbooks and recipe database at dadamo.com and 4yourtype.com.

conducted on practically every patient, resulting in a list of foods to which that person is allergic.

My own patients habitually term any reaction to something they've eaten as a food allergy, although most of the time it is not an allergy they are describing but, rather, a food *intolerance.* If you have a problem with lactose in milk, for example, you are not allergic to it; you lack an enzyme to break it down. You are lactose intolerant, not lactose allergic. This intolerance does not necessarily mean you'll get sick if you drink milk. Type Bs who are lactose intolerant, for example, are often able to gradually introduce small amounts of cultured milk products into their diets. There are also products that add the lactose enzyme to milk products, making them more palatable for the intolerant.

Although the basis of food allergy testing is scientifically valid, sometimes the interpretation is not. Patients have come in with food allergy results that did not show a reaction to foods that they have already had a profound allergic reaction to. Other tests show a food allergy exists, but the patient has eaten the food for years and never had any problems with it. Oftentimes it seems the antibody is being linked to a food protein when in fact it may well be a common protein shared among foods and microbes in the gut.

True food allergies exist, but the effects of a food allergy do not occur in the digestive tract but in the immune system. Your immune system literally creates an antibody to a food. The reaction is swift and harsh—rashes, swelling, cramps, or other specific symptoms that indicate your body is struggling to rid itself of the food it is allergic to.

Food allergies don't just affect the gut. Dietary lectins have been shown to produce immunoglobulin E (IgE), an antibody that triggers allergic reactions, which is why people who follow the Blood Type Diet have a lessening of sinus and asthma symptoms. Each Blood Type Diet is rich in natural antioxidants called flavones, which block specialized cells called basophils from releasing IgE unnecessarily.

Not everything in nature is perfectly cut and dried. Allergic reactions can be genetic, and those genes can be independent of your blood type. Occasionally, I'll come across a person who is allergic to a food that is on his Blood Type Diet. The solution? Simply remove the offending food. The main point is that you have more to fear from the hidden lectins entering your system than you do from food allergies. You may not feel sick when you eat the food, but it is affecting your system nonetheless. Type A should also be aware of excessive mucus production. What may appear to be an allergy is actually the result of eating mucus-producing foods.

### ASTHMA AND HAY FEVER

Type Os win the allergy sweepstakes hands down. They are more likely to suffer from asthma. Even hay fever, the bane of so many, appears to be specific to Type O blood. A wide range of pollens contain lectins that stimulate the release of the powerful histamines, and boom! Itching, sneezing, runny nose, wheezing, coughing, watery eyes—all allergy symptoms.

Many food lectins, especially wheat, interact with IgE antibodies found in the blood. These antibodies stimulate basophils to release not only histamines but other powerful chemical allergens called kinins. These can cause severe allergic reactions, such as swelling in throat tissues and constriction in the lungs.

Asthma and hay fever sufferers do best when they follow the diet recommended for their blood type. For example, a Type O who eliminates wheat and corn often finds relief of many symptoms, such as sneezing, respiratory problems, snoring, and persistent digestive disorders.

Type As have a different problem. Instead of environmental reactions, they often develop stress-related asthma as a result of their stress profile, particularly high cortisol levels. When a Type A suffers from excessive production of mucus caused by poor dietary choices, it makes the stress-related asthma worse. In addition, Type As naturally produce copious amounts of mucus, and when they eat foods that are mucus producing (such as uncultured dairy), they'll have more respiratory problems. When Type A is careful to avoid mucus-producing foods, and when the causes of the stress are addressed positively, the asthmatic condition always improves or is eliminated.

By design, Type B appears to be less prone to developing allergies—unless the wrong foods are eaten. For example, chicken and corn lectins may trigger allergies in even the most resistant Type B.

Type ABs seem to have the least problem with allergies, probably because their immune system is the most environmentally friendly. The combination of A-like and B-like antigens gives Type AB a double dose of antigens with which to deal with environmental intrusion.

## Autoimmune Disorders

Autoimmune disorders are immune-system breakdowns. Your immune defenses develop what amounts to severe amnesia; they no longer recognize themselves. The result is that they run amok, making autoantibodies, which attack their own tissues. These warlike autoantibodies think they are protecting their turf, but in reality they are destroying their own organs and inciting inflammatory responses. Examples of autoimmune disease are rheumatoid arthritis, lupus nephritis, many forms of kidney disease, and possibly elements of chronic fatigue syndrome (Epstein-Barr virus), multiple sclerosis, and amyotrophic lateral sclerosis (ALS, also known as Lou Gehrig's disease).

### Arthritis

My father observed many years ago that Type O tended to develop a gritty sort of arthritis, a chronic deterioration of the bone cartilage. This is the kind of arthritic condition called osteoarthritis, typically found in the elderly. The Type O immune system is environmentally intolerant, and there are many foods—grains and potatoes among them—whose lectins induce inflammatory reactions in the joints. Also, if a Type O individual has had a lifetime of insufficient protein intake, there may be extensive bone demineralization. Remember, Type O needs a reasonable amount of protein and fat in the diet to activate the calcium-absorbing enzyme in the gut.

Type A tends to develop a puffy arthritis, which is the more acute rheumatoid form of the disease—a painful and debilitating breakdown of multiple joints.

In my own practice, most of my patients who suffer from rheumatoid arthritis are Type A. The anomaly of Type A, with its immunological tolerance, developing this form of arthritis may be related to A-specific lectins. Laboratory animals injected with lectins known to react with the A antigen developed inflammation and joint destruction that was indistinguishable from rheumatoid arthritis. Just as likely, there is a stress connection. Some studies show that people with rheumatoid arthritis tend to be more high-strung, more prone to sleep disturbance, and less emotionally hardy. Many of these are the same symptoms of a dysregulated cortisol metabolism, a tendency common in Type A. When Type As have poor coping mechanisms for life stress, the disease progresses more rapidly. This makes some sense in light of what we know about the stress factor and about the risks for Type A. Type A individuals with rheumatoid arthritis should certainly incorporate daily relaxation techniques, as well as calming exercises.

### Chronic Fatigue Syndrome

In recent years, I have treated many people who suffered from the baffling disease called chronic fatigue syndrome (CFS). The primary symptom is great tiredness. Other more advanced symptoms include painful muscles and joints, persistent sore throats, digestive problems, allergies, and chemical sensitivities. The most important thing I've learned from my research and clinical work is that CFS may not be an exclusively autoimmune disease at all, but rather a detoxification issue, caused by poor liver metabolism and the inability to neutralize harmful chemicals. To my reasoning, only this sort of liver problem could produce immunological effects as well as effects characteristic of other systems, such as digestive or musculoskeletal.

I've found that Type O CFS patients in particular do very well on licorice and potassium supplements, in addition to the Blood Type Diet. Licorice has many effects in the body, but in the liver it really shines. The bile ducts, where detoxification occurs, become more efficient, offering greater protection against chemical damage. This preliminary removal of stress to the liver seems to positively influence the adrenals and blood sugar, increasing energy and producing a feeling of well-being. The blood type–specific exercise activities also seem to serve as a valuable guide to help patients return to appropriate forms of physical activity. (Note: Please do not use licorice without a physician's supervision.)

### Case History: Chronic Fatigue Syndrome
*from Dr. John Prentice, Everett, Washington*
Karen, Age 44; Blood Type B

My colleague Dr. John Prentice tried the Blood Type Diet for the first time on a patient with severe CFS. He wasn't totally convinced it would work, but all efforts to help his very sick patient had failed, and he contacted me when he heard of the work I was doing with CFS patients.

Karen was a tough case. She had suffered terrible fatigue for her entire adult life and had needed 12 hours of sleep every night since she was a teenager. She would steal naps when she could. For the past seven years her exhaustion prevented her from holding a job. In addition, her neck, shoulders, and back were constantly in pain, and she suffered debilitating headaches. Recently, Karen had started experiencing terrible anxiety attacks, with heart palpitations so severe she would call 911. It felt as if her circulation was shutting down, along with her whole body.

Karen was a wealthy woman, but most of her inheritance was spent on making the rounds to doctors. She had been to more than 50 doctors, both conventional and alternative, before she came to Dr. Prentice.

Dr. Prentice started Karen on a program of strict adherence to the Type B Diet, supplements, and exercise regimen. Both he and Karen were astonished to see that within only a week she had a tremendous increase in energy. Within a few weeks, most of her symptoms were resolved.

Dr. Prentice tells me that today Karen is a new person. "It's like clockwork," he says. "When she eats 'off' her diet, her body reminds her with severe symptoms, so she sticks with it closely." He shared a letter she had written to him: "I have a whole new life. All my symptoms are practically gone and I hold two jobs, having great energy fourteen hours a day consistently. I believe the diet is key to this tremendous change. I am extremely active and feel like nothing can stop me. Thank you so very much!"

### Multiple Sclerosis, Lou Gehrig's Disease

Both multiple sclerosis (MS) and Lou Gehrig's disease (ALS) appear to be more frequent in Blood Type B. It's an example of the Type B tendency to contract unusual slow-growing viral and neurological disorders. The Type B association may explain why many Jewish populations, which have high percentages of Type B individuals, suffer from these diseases more than other groups. Some researchers believe that multiple sclerosis and Lou Gehrig's disease are caused by a virus, contracted in youth, that has a stealthy B-like appearance. The virus cannot be combated by Type Bs since they do not produce anti-B antibodies. The virus grows slowly and produces no symptoms for 20 or more years. From there it activates the more generalized parts of the immune system to produce inflammation and destruction of the myelin sheathing around nerve cells. Another possibility is that because Type B appears to produce nitric oxide easier than Type O and Type A, the reaction to the causative factors (viral, etc.) may be more intense, leading to greater inflammation and nerve cell death. Type ABs are also at risk for MS and ALS because they share many of the same tendencies regarding the production of nitric oxide.

### Case History: Autoimmune Disorder
### Joan, Age 55; Blood Type O

Joan, a middle-aged dentist's wife, was a classic example of an individual living with the ravages of autoimmune disorders. She suffered from severe symptoms of chronic fatigue/Epstein-Barr, arthritis, and tremendous discomfort caused by gas and bloating. Joan's digestive system was so disrupted that practically everything she ate caused bouts of diarrhea. By the time she arrived in my office, she had been struggling with these conditions for more than a year. Needless to say, she was terribly weakened and in great pain. She was also very discouraged. Because autoimmune disorders can be hard to pin down, many people (even some physicians) don't believe those who suffer from autoimmune diseases like CFS are really sick. Imagine the humiliation and frustration of feeling deathly ill but having people tell you it's all in your head!

Worse still, Joan's doctors had experimented with a number of drug therapies, including steroids, which made her even sicker and contributed to her bloating. She had also been told to adopt a diet high in grains and vegetables, and to limit or eliminate red meat—exactly the opposite of what this Type O should have been doing.

As severe as Joan's symptoms were, the treatment was fairly simple—a detoxification program, the Type O Diet, and a regimen of nutritional supplements. Within two weeks, Joan experienced significant improvement. By the six-month mark, she was feeling normal again. To this day, Joan's energy level is good, her digestion is healthy, and her arthritis flares up only when she binges on carbs and dairy products.

Case History: Lupus
*From Dr. Thomas Kruzel, Gresham, Oregon*
Marcia, Age 30; Blood Type A

My colleague Dr. Kruzel was interested in trying the blood type treatments, but he was initially skeptical. It was a case of lupus nephritis that showed him the true value of serotyping for the treatment of disease.

Marcia, a frail young woman suffering from lupus, was carried into Dr. Kruzel's office by her brother after being discharged from the hospital's intensive care unit. She had suffered kidney failure from circulating immune complexes related to her disease. Marcia had been on shunt dialysis for several weeks and was scheduled for renal transplantation within the next six months.

Dr. Kruzel took her history and learned that Marcia's diet was very high in dairy, wheat, and red meat—all dangerous foods for a Type A person in her condition. He placed her on a strict vegetarian diet along with hydrotherapy and homeopathic preparations. Within two weeks, Marcia's condition had improved and her need for dialysis had decreased. Remarkably, within a two-month period, Marcia was taken completely off dialysis and her previously scheduled kidney transplant was canceled.

## Blood Disorders

It should come as no surprise that blood-related illnesses, such as anemia and clotting disorders, are blood type specific.

### Pernicious Anemia

Type A makes up the greatest number of pernicious anemia sufferers, but the condition has nothing to do with the vegetarian Type A Diet. Pernicious anemia is the result of a vitamin $B_{12}$ deficiency, and Type A has the most difficulty absorbing $B_{12}$ from food. Type AB also has a tendency toward pernicious anemia, although not as great as Type A.

The reason for the deficiency is that the body's use of vitamin $B_{12}$ requires high levels of stomach acid and the presence of intrinsic factor, a chemical produced by the lining of the stomach that is responsible for the vitamin's assimilation. Type A and Type AB have lower levels of intrinsic factor than the other blood types and don't produce as much stomach acid. For this reason, most Type As and Type ABs who suffer from pernicious anemia respond best when vitamin $B_{12}$ is administered by injection. By eliminating the need for the digestive process to assimilate this vital and potent nutrient, it is made available to the body in a more highly concentrated way. This is a case in which dietary solutions alone don't work, although Type A and Type AB are able to absorb Floradix, a liquid iron and herb supplement.

Given a proper diet, Type O and Type B tend not to suffer from anemia; they have high acid contents in their stomachs and sufficient levels of intrinsic factor.

### Case History: Anemia

*From Dr. Jonathan V. Wright, Kent, Washington*

Carol, Age 35; Blood Type O

My colleague Dr. Jonathan Wright successfully used the Blood Type Diet to treat a woman with chronically low blood levels of iron. Carol had tried every available form of iron supplement with no success, and Dr. Wright had tried a number of other treatments also without success. The only thing that worked at all was injectable iron, but that was only a temporary solution. Her iron levels would inevitably drop again.

I had talked to Dr. Wright on an earlier occasion about my work with lectins and blood types, and he called me for more details. He decided to try the Blood Type O Diet for Carol. After eliminating the incompatible lectins, which may have been damaging her red blood cells, and adhering to a high–animal protein diet, Carol improved; her blood iron levels started to rise and the previously ineffective supplementation started to help. Dr. Wright and I agreed that the agglutination of the intestinal tract by the incompatible food lectins prevented the iron from assimilating.

### Clotting Disorders

Type O faces the biggest problems when it comes to blood clotting. Most often, Type O lacks sufficient quantities of the various blood-clotting factors. This can have severe consequences, especially during surgery or in situations where there is blood loss. Type O women, for example, tend to lose significantly more blood after childbirth than women of other blood types.

Type Os with a history of bleeding disorders and stroke should emphasize foods containing chlorophyll to help modify their clotting factors. Chlorophyll is found in almost all green vegetables and also can be taken as a supplement.

In studies, Type A and Type AB individuals tend to predominate with clotting disorders, and their thicker blood can work to their disadvantage in other ways. Thicker blood is more likely to induce inflammation in the arteries—one reason Type A and AB are more prone to cardiovascular diseases. Type A and Type AB women might have problems with heavy clotting during menstrual periods if they don't keep their diets under control. Several diseases have been shown to increase the already high blood viscosity (thickness) in Type A and AB individuals, including cancer, diabetes, peripheral artery disease and stress—another reason to practice targeted stress reduction techniques such as yoga and tai chi.

Type Bs tend not to suffer from clotting disorders or thick blood. As long as they follow the Blood Type B Diet, their balanced systems work efficiently.

## Cardiovascular Disease

Cardiovascular disease is epidemic in Western societies, with many factors to blame, including diet, lack of exercise, smoking, and stress.

Is there a connection between your blood type and your susceptibility to cardiovascular disease? When researchers associated with the famous Framingham [Massachusetts] Heart Study examined the connection between blood type and heart disease, they found no clear-cut blood type distinction in terms of who gets heart disease. They did, however, discover a strong connection between blood type and who survives heart disease. The study found that Type O heart patients between the ages of 39 and 72 had a much higher rate of survival than Type A heart patients in the same age group. This was especially true for men between the ages of 50 and 59.

Although the Framingham Heart Study did not explore this subject in real depth, it appears that the same factors involved in surviving heart disease also offer some protection against developing it in the first place. While Type A and Type AB have a higher risk for cardiovascular disease, in general, research and clinical practice also show that the pathway to cardiovascular disease differs depending on your blood type.

High cholesterol is more likely to be a high risk factor for coronary artery disease for Type A and Type AB. Most of the cholesterol in our bodies is produced in our livers, but there is an enzyme called phosphatase manufactured in the small intestine that is responsible for the absorption of dietary fats. High alkaline phosphatase levels, which speed the absorption and metabolism of fats, lead to low serum cholesterol levels. Type O blood normally has the highest natural levels of this enzyme, followed by Type B. Type AB and Type A have lower levels of alkaline phosphatase enzyme. Type A and, to a slightly lesser extent, Type AB have consistently higher levels of serum cholesterol and triglycerides (blood fats) than do Type O and Type B blood. In this case, Type O's "thin" blood, the result of fewer blood clotting factors, is actually protective against plaque deposits.

That is not to say that Blood Types O and B don't have risk factors for cardiovascular disease. Diets high in carbohydrates lead to insulin resistance, obesity, and high triglycerides. Increasing evidence shows that high triglycerides are as great a risk factor for heart disease as high cholesterol. Certain stress profiles, such as the "Type A personality," characterized by excessive anger, anxiety, and aggression, have been associated with a greater incidence of heart disease. As we've discovered, it is rather ironic that such behavior is in fact associated with

Type O blood. Progressive and strenuous exercise is the best way for Type Os to bulletproof themselves against heart disease.

### CASE HISTORY: HEART DISEASE
### WILMA, AGE 52; BLOOD TYPE O

Wilma was a 52-year-old Lebanese woman with advanced cardiovascular disease. When I first examined her, she had recently come out of the hospital after receiving a balloon angioplasty, a procedure used to treat clogged coronary arteries.

Since Wilma was Type O, I was fairly certain that her problem was mainly dietary.

Wilma had always eaten the traditional Lebanese diet, including lots of grains and fish. However, five years earlier, she began to experience pain in her neck and arms. Heart disease didn't even occur to her! She assumed the pain was arthritis and was stunned when her doctor diagnosed her problem as angina pectoris, pain caused from an inadequate blood and oxygen supply to the heart muscle.

After her angioplasty, Wilma's cardiologist advised her to begin taking a statin to lower cholesterol. A well-read health consumer, Wilma worried about long-term problems with drug therapy, and she wanted to try a natural approach before opting for the drug. That's when she came to me.

Since Wilma was Type O, I suggested that she add lean red meat to her diet. In light of her condition, she was understandably nervous about eating foods that are usually restricted in people with high cholesterol or heart disease. She immediately consulted her cardiologist, who was—no surprise—appalled at the idea. Again, he urged her to take the statin medication. But Wilma was serious about avoiding drug therapy, so she decided to follow the Blood Type O Diet for three months and do a cholesterol check at that time.

Wilma confirmed many of my theories about susceptibility to high cholesterol. Often, through heredity or by other mechanisms, people have high levels of cholesterol in their blood in spite of a severely restricted diet. Usually they have some defect in the manipulation of the internal cholesterol metabolism. My suspicion is that when Type O individuals eat a lot of certain carbohydrates (usually wheat products), it modifies the effectiveness of their insulin, resulting in its becoming more potent and longer lasting. From the increased insulin activity, the body stores more fat in the tissues and elevates the triglyceride stores.

In addition to advising Wilma to increase the percentage of red meat in her diet, I also helped her find substitutes for the large amounts of wheat she was consuming and prescribed an extract of hawthorn (an herb used as a tonic for the heart and arteries) and a low dose of the B vitamin niacin (which helps reduce cholesterol levels).

Wilma was an executive secretary with a stressful job, and she did very little exercise. She was intrigued when I described the relationship between stress and physical activity in people with Type O blood as well as the relationship between stress and heart disease. She had never been a regular exerciser, so hardly knew where to begin. I started her on a walking program to gradually increase her aerobic fitness. After a couple of weeks, Wilma reported that walking was a godsend; she'd never felt better.

Within six months Wilma's cholesterol plummeted, without medication, to 187, where it stabilized. She was elated to have cholesterol in the normal range. It had seemed impossible.

The naturopath intern working in my office was astounded and perplexed. All conventional evidence indicates that people with high cholesterol should avoid red meats, yet Wilma flourished. Blood type was the missing link.

### CASE HISTORY: DANGEROUSLY HIGH CHOLESTEROL
### JOHN, AGE 23; BLOOD TYPE O

John, a recent college graduate, had a skyrocketing cholesterol level, high triglycerides, and high blood sugar. These were very unusual symptoms for a young man, but as there was a strong family history of heart disease, naturally his parents were alarmed. After extensive workups at Yale by consulting cardiologists, John was told that his genetic predisposition was so overwhelming that even cholesterol-reducing medication would be useless. In effect, John was told that he was destined to develop coronary artery disease—sooner, rather than later.

In the office, John seemed depressed and lethargic. He complained of severe fatigue. "I used to love to work out," he said, "but now I just don't have the energy." John also suffered from frequent sore throats and swollen glands. His past history revealed mononucleosis and two separate incidences of Lyme disease.

John had been following a vegetarian diet prescribed by his cardiologist for some time. He admitted, however, that he was feeling worse on this diet, not better.

After only a few weeks on the Blood Type O Diet, however, the results were amazing. Within five months, John's serum cholesterol, triglycerides, and blood sugar all dropped to normal levels. A repeat blood profile after three months revealed similar results.

If John continues to follow the Blood Type O Diet, exercise regularly, and take nutritional supplements, there is a good chance that he will beat the odds of his genetic inheritance.

Constantly at work within us is the dynamic force of our beating hearts, rhythmically pumping blood through our bodies. The process is normally so smooth that we rarely think much about it. That's why high blood pressure (or hypertension) is called the silent killer. It's possible to have dangerously high blood pressure and be entirely unaware of it.

When blood pressure is taken, two numbers are read. The systolic reading (the number on top) measures the pressure within the arteries as your heart beats out blood. The diastolic reading (the number on the bottom) measures the pressure present within the arteries as your heart rests between beats. Normal systolic pressure is below 120, and normal diastolic pressure is below 80. Elevated blood pressure is any number above 120/80, with high blood pressure (or hypertension) at 140/90.

Depending on the severity and duration, high blood pressure left untreated opens the door to a host of problems, including heart attacks and strokes. Hypertension often occurs in conjunction with heart disease, so Type A and Type AB should be particularly vigilant. Hypertension carries the same risk factors as cardiovascular disease. Smokers, diabetics, postmenopausal women, the obese, the sedentary, and people in stressful positions should pay extra attention to the details of their Blood Type Diet.

### CASE HISTORY: HYPERTENSION
### BILL, AGE 54; BLOOD TYPE A

Bill was a middle-aged bond trader with high blood pressure. When I first saw him in my office, his blood pressure was an almost explosive 150/105 to 135/95. It didn't take me long to find clues to these numbers in his incredibly stressful life, which included a partnership in a high-powered firm and a host of domestic problems. Against his doctor's urging, Bill had discontinued his blood pressure medication because it made him dizzy and constipated. He wanted to try a more natural therapy, but it had to be done immediately.

I placed Bill on a Blood Type A Diet—a huge adjustment for this burly Italian-American. And I immediately began to address Bill's stress with the exercise regimen designed for Type As. He was initially embarrassed about doing yoga and relaxation exercises, but was soon converted when he saw how much calmer and more positive he felt.

At his first visit, Bill also confided that he had a special problem of a different nature. He and his partners were in the process of negotiating their office health plan, and if his hypertension were detected at his insurance physical, his firm would have to pay a much higher premium. Using the stress-reduction techniques, the Blood Type A Diet, and several botanicals, Bill was able to sail through his insurance physical.

Paradoxically, throughout Bill's treatment his insurance company refused to reimburse him for naturopathic care, claiming that it was not a medical necessity. When presented with his now-lower blood pressure readings, they claimed that his company would still have to pay the higher premiums because his condition was being medically treated! As he tells it, Bill went all the way to the president of the insurance company and said, "Look, you can't have it both ways—refuse to pay for the treatment and then claim that the same treatment is the reason why our premiums must remain high." He got his company's premium reduced that afternoon, and the next day the insurance company president scheduled an appointment at our clinic.

## Childhood Illnesses

A large number of the patients who come through my office are children suffering from a host of ailments—from chronic diarrhea to repeated ear infections. Their mothers are usually on the verge of frantic. Some of my most satisfying results have come with children.

### Conjunctivitis

Conjunctivitis, commonly called "pink eye," is usually caused by the transmission of the staphylococcus bacteria from one child to another. Type A and Type AB children are more susceptible to conjunctivitis than are Type O or Type B, probably because of their weaker immune systems.

Antibiotic creams or eyedrops are used to treat the condition in the conventional manner. But a soothing and surprising alternative is a freshly cut slice of tomato. (Don't try this with tomato juice!) The freshly cut tomato contains a lectin that can agglutinate and destroy the staphylococcus bacteria. The slight acidity of the tomato appears to resemble closely the acidity of the eye's own secretions. Squeezing the watery juice of a fresh tomato on a gauze pad and applying it to the affected eye is also very soothing.

This is one example of how the same lectins in a food that make it dangerous to eat can be highly beneficial to treat an illness. Later, we'll discuss many other examples of the ways in which lectins play a dual role—good cop, bad cop—in our systems. Especially in the war against cancer.

### Diarrhea

Diarrhea can be a disturbing and dangerous condition for children. Not only is it debilitating and terribly uncomfortable but it can lead to severe dehydration, causing weakness and fever.

Most childhood diarrhea is the result of either microbial imbalance or dietary irregularities, and here the Blood Type Diet offers very specific guidelines about which foods trigger digestive problems for each blood type.

Type O children often experience mild to moderate diarrhea, frequently caused by the milder forms of coliform bacteria. This often results from an overreliance on dairy products or an excessive use of grains and carbs due to the child's picky eating habits.

Type A and Type AB children are prone to *Giardia lamblia*, more commonly known as Montezuma's revenge. The giardia parasite mimics the Blood Type A antigen and can evade a proper immune response.

Type B children will often contract diarrhea if they overindulge in wheat products or in reaction to eating chicken and corn. If they are Type B secretors (about 80 percent of all Type Bs), they may have a problem with the norovirus, a very common cause of diarrhea.

If the diarrhea is caused by food-related intolerance or allergy, your child will often exhibit other symptoms, ranging from dark, puffy circles under the eyes to eczema, psoriasis, or asthma.

Unless diarrhea is the result of a more serious condition, such as a parasitic infection, partial intestinal blockage, or inflammation, it usually corrects itself with time. Should your child's stool contain blood or mucus, however, seek immediate medical attention. Acute diarrhea might also be infectious; to protect the rest of your family from contagion, it is best to institute scrupulous standards of cleanliness.

To restore your child's proper balance of fluids during bouts of diarrhea, restrict fruit juice. Instead, feed your child vegetable or meat stocks in soups. One wonderful herb that can be used for all blood types is carob. Not only is carob effective for simple cases of diarrhea but it has a wonderful chocolate-like taste that kids really enjoy.

### EAR INFECTIONS

Perhaps as many as two-thirds of children under the age of six have chronic ear infections. By chronic, I mean 5, 10, 15, even 20 infections every winter season, one after the other. Most of these children have allergies to both environmental and food-based particles. The best solution is the Blood Type Diet.

The conventional protocol for ear infections is antibiotic therapy, but it obviously fails when there is a chronic infection. If we attack the underlying causes of the problem first instead of trotting out the most currently fashionable nostrum—and by this I mean the ever more sophisticated and newest classes of antibiotics—we have an opportunity to allow the body to mount its own powerful response. For starters, it is helpful to know the blood type susceptibilities.

Children who are Type A and Type AB have greater problems with mucus secretions from improper diet—a factor in ear infections. In Type A children, dairy products are usually the culprit, whereas Type AB may experience sensitivities to corn in addition to milk. In general, these kids are also more likely to have throat and respiratory problems, which can often move into the ears. Because the immune systems of Type A and Type AB children are tolerant of a wider range of bacteria, some of their problems stem from the lack of an aggressive response to the infectious organism. Several studies have shown that ear fluids of children with a history of chronic ear infections lack specific chemicals called complement, which are needed to attack and destroy the bacteria.

Another study shows that a serum lectin called mannose-binding protein is missing in the ear fluids of children with chronic infections. This lectin apparently binds to mannose sugars on the surface of the bacteria and agglutinates them, allowing for their faster removal. Both of these important immune factors eventually develop in their proper amounts, which may help explain why the frequency of ear infections gradually lessens as the child ages. In addition to diet, treating Type A and Type AB children with ear infections almost always involves enhancing their immunity. The simplest way to enhance the immunity of any child is to cut down on their intake of sugar. Numerous studies have shown that sugar depresses the immune system, making the body's white blood cells sluggish and disinclined to attack invading organisms.

Naturopaths have for many years made use of a mild herbal immune stimulant, *Echinacea purpurea*. Originally used by Native Americans, echinacea has the extraordinary properties of being both safe and effective in boosting the body's immunity against bacteria and viruses. Because many of the immune functions that echinacea enhances depend on adequate levels of vitamin C, I often prescribe an extract of vitamin C–rich rose hips. In my experience, echinacea preparations seem to work better for Types A, B, and AB than they do for Type O. I also use an extract of the western larch tree as a sort of super-echinacea. This product, larch arabinogalactan, contains much more concentrated active components than you get with echinacea.

Ear infections are terribly painful for a child, and not too pleasant for the parents either. Most of these infections are a backup of noxious fluids and gases into the middle ear because of an obstructed connecting pipe, the eustachian tube. This tube can become swollen because of allergic reactions, weakness in the tissues surrounding it, or infections.

Many parents have grown frustrated by the increasing inability of antibiotics to work on ear infections. There is a reason for this resistance: A baby's first ear infection is typically treated with a mild antibiotic, such as amoxicillin. With the child's next ear infection, amoxicillin is given again. Eventually, the ever more resistant infection returns, and amoxicillin is no longer effective. The escalation phenomenon—the process of using stronger and stronger drugs and ever more invasive treatments—has begun.

When antibiotics no longer work, and the painful infections continue, a myringotomy is performed. This is a process in which tiny tubes called grommets are surgically implanted through the eardrum to increase the drainage of fluid from the middle ear into the throat.

We are now at the point at which most pediatric medical associations are recommending that simple cases of ear infection not be treated with antibiotics at all; instead, they suggest that patients be given supportive care for the pain and a course of antihistamines to help remove the swelling and pressure, something naturopathic physicians have been doing for decades. When I treat chronic ear infections, I focus on ways to prevent recurrences. It is useless to try to resolve one episode with a quick dose of antibiotics when you know another ear infection is warming up in the bull pen. Almost always, I find a solution in the diet.

I see many children in my practice, representing all blood types. I've found that any child can contract chronic ear infections if he eats foods that react poorly in his system. I have never seen a case where there wasn't an obvious connection with a child's favorite food.

Type O and Type B children seem to develop ear infections less frequently, and when they do occur, they are usually easier to treat. More often than not, a change in diet is sufficient to eliminate the problem.

In Type B children, the culprit is usually a viral infection that then leads to a bacterial infection with haemophilus, to which Type B is unusually susceptible. The dietary fix involves restricting tomatoes, corn, and chicken. The lectins in these foods react with the surface of the digestive tract, causing swelling and mucus secretion, which usually carries over to the ears and throat.

My personal feeling is that ear infections can be prevented in Type O children simply by breast-feeding instead of bottle feeding. Breast-feeding for a period of six months to a year allows a child's immune system and digestive tract time to develop. Type O kids will also avoid ear infections if they are taken off wheat and dairy products. They're unusually sensitive to these foods at an early age, but their immunity is easily augmented by the use of higher value proteins such as fish and lean red meats.

Dietary changes are often difficult in households with children who suffer repeated ear infections. Their misery can tempt the anxious parent to let them eat whatever they wish, thinking that it will comfort them. Many of these kids wind up being picky eaters, eating only a very narrow range of foods, and often the very foods that are provoking their illness!

### Case History: Ear Infection
### Tony, Age 7; Blood Type B

Tony was a seven-year-old boy who suffered from repeated ear infections. When his mother first brought him to my office, she was frantic. Tony would develop a new ear infection immediately after stopping the antibiotic used to treat his previous infection, at the rate of 10 to 15 per winter season. He'd had grommet treatment twice, to no avail. This was a perfect example of a child on the antibiotic treadmill: escalating levels of antibiotics with fewer results.

My initial questions to Tony's mother were about his diet. She was a bit defensive. "Oh, I don't think that's the problem," she told me. "We eat very well—lots of chicken and fish, fruits and vegetables."

I turned to Tony. "What are your favorite foods?" I asked.

"Chicken nuggets," he replied enthusiastically.

"Do you like corn on the cob?"

"Oh, yes!"

strain containing a lectin from the edible snail, *Helix aspersa/pomatia.* They reported a strong association between the uptake of the snail lectin and the subsequent development of metastasis to the lymph nodes. In other words, antigens on the surface of the primary breast cancer cells were changing, and this change was allowing the cancer to spread into the lymph nodes. Now, here comes the punch line: The lectin of *Helix aspersa/pomatia* is highly specific—to Blood Type A.

The researchers studying breast cancer discovered that as the cancer cells changed, they made themselves more A-like. This allowed them to bypass all of the body's defenses and rage unimpeded into the defenseless lymph.

Did my Type O patients survive because they were Type O? Did my Type B patients survive because they were Type B? It certainly looked that way.

And there is a confirmation in our scientific understanding of cancer. Many tumor cells have unique antigens, or markers, on their surfaces. For instance, breast cancer patients often show high levels of cancer antigen 15-3 (CA15-3), a marker for breast cancer; ovarian cancer patients often have high levels of CA125; and prostate cancer patients may have an elevated prostate-specific antigen (PSA). These antigens, called tumor markers, are often used to track the progress of the disease and effectiveness of treatment. Many tumor markers possess blood type activity. Sometimes the tumor markers are incomplete or corrupted blood type antigens, which in a normal cell would have gone on to form a part of a person's blood type system.

It is not surprising that many of these tumor markers have A-like qualities, which allow them easy access to the Type A and Type AB systems. There they are welcomed as self—the ultimate molecular Trojan horse. Obviously, the A-like intruders would be more easily detected and eliminated if they were to slip into a Type O or Type B system.

Many breast cancer markers are surprisingly A-like. That's the answer to my question about the differing rates of recurrence on the part of my patients. Although my Type O and Type B patients developed breast cancer, their anti-A antigens were better able to fight it off, rounding up the early cancer cells and destroying them. My Type A and Type AB patients, however, couldn't fight the cancer as well because their systems couldn't see their opponents. Everywhere they turned, the cells looked just like them—and they were unable to detect the mutated cancer cells beneath their clever masks.

### CASE HISTORY: PREVENTING BREAST CANCER
### ANNE, AGE 47; BLOOD TYPE A

Anne came to the office for a general wellness visit, without any real physical complaints. But while I was doing her medical history, I learned that Anne's family had a high incidence of breast cancer on both her mother's and father's sides, and the mortality rate among those who had the disease was very high.

Anne knew about her genetic risk factors, but she was surprised to learn that her Type A blood presented an additional risk factor. "I don't suppose it makes any difference, though," she said. "Either I'm going to get breast cancer or I'm not. There's nothing I can really do about it."

I advised Anne that there were several measures she could take. First, because of her family history, she needed to be hypervigilant about suspicious breast lumps, perform frequent breast self-examinations, and make sure to get routine mammograms.

"When was your last mammogram?" I asked. Anne sheepishly told me that her last mammogram had been seven years before. It turned out that Anne was strongly disinclined to avail herself of any conventional medical techniques. She had educated herself about herbs and vitamins and often used them to treat herself effectively. But when it came to more intrusive medical treatments, she shied away. However, she did promise to schedule a mammogram.

Anne's mammogram was clean, and she began a concentrated program of cancer avoidance. The Blood Type A Diet was an easy transition for Anne because she already ate a primarily vegetarian diet. I fine-tuned the diet with anti-cancer foods, especially increasing the amount of soy and adding specific naturopathic herbs. Anne began to study yoga. She told me that for the first time in her adult life, she wasn't constantly worrying about cancer.

A year later, Anne had a second mammogram. This time a suspicious mark was detected in her left breast. A biopsy showed it to be a precancerous condition known as neoplasia. Essentially, neoplasia is the presence of mutated cells. It's not cancer, but it can become cancer if the cells continue to deteriorate and multiply. During the biopsy, Anne's doctor completely removed the precancerous tissue.

Over the years, there have been no new growths detected, although we watch Anne very carefully. She continues to follow the Blood Type A Diet religiously and says she has never felt healthier.

Of all the functions a physician can perform, none is more elegant and valuable than successful prediction and intervention. I was glad Anne came to me when she did, and that she took all the right steps.

## Immunotherapy

Breast cancer continues to be baffling and too often deadly, but there are some signs that blood type may represent a key to the cure. Immunotherapy is the most promising area of study in fighting all cancers, including breast cancer. There are currently a multitude of clinical trials examining the efficacy of vaccine treatment for cancer. It's a promising direction. One of the early pioneers of this approach used blood type as his basis in creating a vaccine.

The late Georg Springer, a research scientist with the Bligh Cancer Center at the University of Chicago School of Medicine, investigated the effects of a vaccine whose basis is a molecule called the T antigen. Since the 1950s, Springer had been one of the most important investigators in the role of blood type in disease. His contributions to the field were phenomenal, and his work on the T antigen was most promising.

The T antigen is a common tumor marker (pancarcinoma antigen) found in many cancers, especially breast cancer. It shares some similarity with the antigen against Blood Type A. Healthy, cancer-free people carry antibodies against the T antigen, so it is never seen in them. In fact anti-T antibodies are one of the few antibodies that you carry against yourself, although it has been shown that if you are Blood Type A you manufacture less of the antibody than the other blood types. The structure of the T antigen was discovered in the early 1960s by Gerhard Uhlenbruck at the University of Cologne using the lectin from peanuts.

Springer believed that a vaccine composed of the T antigen and several helper molecules called adjuvants could jolt and then reawaken the suppressed immune systems of cancer patients, helping them attack and destroy the cancerous cells. Springer and his colleagues used a vaccine derived from the T antigen, hot-rodded with another common vaccine against typhoid, as a long-term treatment against the recurrence of advanced breast cancer. Although the study group was small—fewer than 25 women—the results are impressive. All of the 11 breast cancer patients who had severely advanced disease (stage III and stage IV) survived for more than five years—remarkable in what is considered end-stage cancer—and 6 of those patients survived more than 10 years. These results are nothing short of miraculous.

Springer's work on blood type systems and cancer convinced me that the natural evolution of our understanding of blood types will eventually provide not just information on risk factors, but also a cure for every manifestation of the disease. Unfortunately Springer's work languished after his death, but I'm happy to report that there has been a considerable surge in research interest in the T antigen in recent years.

There are other ways that blood type may influence the course and outcome of breast cancer. One mechanism involves a molecule called vascular endothelial growth factor (VEGF), which is involved in the development of our vascular network, a process known as angiogenesis. Some evidence suggests that there may be a direct interaction between the Blood Type A antigen and the receptor for VEGF that perhaps could lead to increased production of blood vessels, a process that can help the spread of cancer cells. There is even noncancer evidence of this link: VEGF is responsible for the growth of large birthmarks called port wine stains (hemangiomas), whose occurrence is also known to be more common in Type A individuals.

## Other Forms of Cancer

THE PATHOLOGY of cancer—wild marauders out for a night on the town—is fundamentally the same in all variations, but differences related both to cause and to blood type exist. The A-like or B-like tumor markers exert remarkable control over the way the body's immune system reacts to the cancer's invasion and growth.

Again, almost all cancers show a preference for Type A and Type AB individuals, although there are occasional forms that are B-like, such as female reproductive and bladder cancers. Type O seems to be far more resistant to developing almost any cancer. I believe the intolerant and hostile Type O system, with its more simple fucose sugars, has an easier time tossing off the A-like or B-like cancer cells and developing anti-A or anti-B antibodies.

Again, we unfortunately know little about the full implications of the blood type link in cancers other than breast cancer. However, they most likely follow a similar course. Let's examine some of the most common forms of cancer.

BRAIN TUMORS. Most cancers of the brain and nervous system, such as glioma multiforme and astrocytoma, show a preference for Type A and Type AB individuals. Their tumor markers are A-like.

FEMALE REPRODUCTIVE CANCERS. Cancers of the female reproductive system (uterine, cervical, ovarian, and labial) show a preference for Type A and Type AB. However, there is also a numerically high number of Type B women who suffer from these cancers. This implies there are different tumor markers created, depending on the circumstances. Ovarian cysts and uterine fibroids, which are usually benign but may be a sign of susceptibility to cancer, generate copious amounts of Type A and Type B antigens.

COLON CANCER. Blood type is not the strongest determinant for the various forms of colon cancer. The real risk factors for the conditions that lead to colon cancer are related to diet, lifestyle, and temperament. Ulcerative colitis, Crohn's disease, and irritable bowel syndrome left unmitigated eventually leave the system depleted and open to cancer. A high-fat diet, combined with smoking and alcohol consumption, create the ideal environment for digestive cancers. The risk is greater if you have a family history of colon cancer. That said, Type A and Type AB individuals are at higher risk.

MOUTH AND UPPER DIGESTIVE CANCERS. Cancers of the lip, tongue, gums, and cheek; tumors of the salivary gland; and esophageal cancer are all strongly linked to Type A and Type AB blood. Most of these cancers are self-generated, in that the risks can be minimized if you abstain from tobacco, moderate your alcohol consumption, and watch your diet.

STOMACH AND ESOPHAGEAL CANCER. Stomach cancer is attracted to low levels of stomach acid, a Type A and Type AB trait. In well over 63,000 cases of stomach cancer studied, Type A and Type AB were predominant. Stomach cancer is epidemic in China, Japan, and Korea because the typical diet is rich in smoked, pickled, and fermented foods. These Asian dietary staples seem to counter any of the good that soybeans might do, perhaps because they are packed with carcinogenic nitrates. Asian Type Bs, who have higher levels of stomach acid, aren't as prone to stomach cancer, even if they eat some of the same foods.

PANCREATIC, LIVER, GALLBLADDER, AND BILE DUCT CANCERS. Cancers of the pancreas, liver, and gallbladder are rare in Type O, with its hardy digestive systems. A study by the Dana-Farber Cancer Institute showed that people with Blood Types A, B, and AB were more likely to develop pancreatic cancer than Type Os. Type A and Type AB are at most risk; Type B has some susceptibility, especially when consuming certain nuts and seeds that are unsuitable.

Several of the earlier therapies for these cancers included large portions of fresh liver from sheep, horse, and buffalo. They seemed to help, but no one knew why. It was later discovered that the livers of these animals contained lectins that slowed the growth and spread of pancreatic, liver, gallbladder, and bile duct cancers.

CASE HISTORY: LIVER CANCER
CATHY, AGE 49; BLOOD TYPE A

Cathy first sought medical attention for a suspicious growth in her abdomen, which turned out to be an aggressive form of liver cancer. She was treated at Harvard's Deaconess Hospital in Boston, Massachusetts, and eventually received a liver transplant. She was referred to me two years later.

In the subsequent two years, most of my focus was on using naturopathic techniques to replace the immunosuppressing antirejection drugs needed to help her keep her transplanted liver. Cathy's condition improved to the point that she was able to stop her drug therapy.

However, after two years of this protocol, Cathy was experiencing some shortness of breath, and at her checkup at Harvard, doctors noticed suspicious lesions on a chest X-ray. These turned out to be cancer.

Cathy and her physicians were on the horns of a dilemma. Her lungs were so heavily laced with cancer, surgery was out of the question ("It would be like picking cherries," said her surgeon), and her liver transplant ruled out chemotherapy.

We went to work, using the basic Type A–lectin cancer diet and other immune-enhancing botanicals. I also recommended a preparation made from shark cartilage for Cathy to take orally and use as an enema.

In an amazing series of correspondences, Cathy's surgical team at Harvard kept me up-to-date on her progress, including informing me that the lesions in Cathy's lungs had shrunk and looked more like scar tissue. Subsequent letters confirmed these findings. In time even the scar tissue began to disappear.

Cathy was stunned and overjoyed. "When they told me that the cancer seemed to be going into remission, I felt as if I had won the lottery," she said happily. Cathy went on to live three symptom-free years. Unfortunately, her cancer finally returned, and she later died.

The case is especially interesting for two reasons: First, throughout this time Cathy received no treatment other than naturopathic. Second, her team at Harvard was open-minded about and supportive of her using a naturopathic doctor. Perhaps what we have seen here is a tiny glimpse of the future: all medical systems working together for the betterment of the patient.

By the way, the total cost of Cathy's naturopathic therapy was less than $1,500, as opposed to the tens of thousands she might have spent on conventional treatment.

Lymphomas, Leukemias, and Hodgkin's Disease. Type O may be predisposed to lymphomas, leukemias, and Hodgkin's disease.

Although these diseases of the blood and lymph preferentially afflict Type O, they may not be true cancers at all, but rather viral infections that have run amok. This would make some sense in light of what we know about Type Os; they're actually pretty good at fighting most cancers, but the Type O antigen is not well designed for fighting viruses.

LUNG CANCER. Lung cancer is truly nonspecific. It is one of the few cancers that has no particular blood type connection. Lung cancer is most commonly caused by cigarette smoking. Yes, lung cancer is caused by many other things as well. There are people who have never smoked who will die of lung cancer as you are reading this sentence. But we all know that smoking is the overwhelming cause of lung cancer. Tobacco is such a powerful carcinogen in its own right that it bypasses anything so obvious and so ordered as predilection.

PROSTATE CANCER. There appears to be a higher level of prostate cancer in secretors. My own experience has been that a greater number of Type A and Type AB men suffer from prostate cancer than do Type O or Type B men. A Type A or Type AB secretor is at the highest risk.

SKIN AND BONE CANCERS. Type A and Type AB individuals are at greatest risk for malignant melanoma, the deadliest form of skin cancer, although Type O and Type B are not immune. Bone cancers seem to show a consistent preference for Type B, although there is some risk for Type A and Type AB individuals.

URINARY TRACT, KIDNEY, AND BLADDER CANCERS. Bladder cancer in both men and women occurs most often in Type A and Type B individuals. Type ABs, who have the double whammy of both A and B characteristics, are probably at the greatest risk of all. Far more than Type A, Type B individuals who suffer from recurrent bladder and kidney infections should be especially careful with the management of this problem, as it inevitably leads to more serious diseases. One puzzling connection that is yet to be unraveled: Wheat germ agglutinin, the lectin that can act favorably against both lobular and intraductal breast cancers, paradoxically accelerates the growth of bladder cancer cells.

## Fighting Back

Cancer always seems to present a discouraging picture. I imagine that if you are Type A or Type AB, you may be thinking grim thoughts. Remember, though, that susceptibility is a single factor among many. I believe that knowing your predilection for cancer and understanding the workings of your specific blood type gives you more opportunity than you would otherwise have to fight back. The following strategies provide a way to make a difference for yourself, especially if you are Type A or Type AB. In particular, many of the foods suggested are tailored for these blood types. Current research has focused primarily on the A-like markers for breast cancer, and little investigation has been conducted regarding the B-like cancers. Unfortunately, this means that while the cancer-fighting foods suggested here may be very effective for Type A and Type AB, they won't necessarily help Type B or Type O. In fact, most of these foods (peanuts, soy, lentils, and wheat germ) cause other problems for the latter two blood types.

Continued research will one day give us a deeper understanding of the cancer-diet connection for all the blood types. In the meantime, here are some special recommendations for people with Type A and AB.

### You Live as You Eat

People with Type A blood have digestive tracts that find it difficult to break down animal fats and proteins. Type A and Type AB should adhere to a diet high in fiber and low in animal products.

There are specific foods that must be given extra consideration as cancer preventives.

### Soybeans . . . Again

Between 3 and 11 percent of every cake of tofu is composed of soybean agglutinins. Soybean agglutinins are able to selectively identify early mutated cells producing the Type A antigen and sweep them from the system, leaving normal Type A cells alone. Although soy foods are a rich source, only a minute amount is needed for agglutination.

The soybean agglutinin especially discriminates when it comes to breast cancer cells; it is so specific that it's been used to remove cancerous cells from harvested bone marrow. In experimental work breast cancer patients had their bone marrow removed and were then bombarded with high levels of chemotherapy and radiation. These oncology tools would normally destroy the bone marrow. Instead, the harvested marrow—cleansed by soybean lectin—was then reintroduced into the patients. These treatments have shown some very good results.

The soybean lectin also contains estrogen-related compounds genistein and daidzein. These compounds not only help balance the effect of a woman's estrogen levels but also contain other properties that can help reduce the blood supply to tumor cells.

Soybeans in all forms are beneficial to Type A and Type AB as a general cancer preventative. The vegetable proteins in soy are easier for these blood types to use, and so it is strongly suggested that these blood types reexamine any aversion they may have to tofu and tofu products. Think of tofu not only as a food, but as a powerful medicine.

Japanese women have such a low incidence of breast cancer because the use of tofu and other soy products is still high in the overall Japanese diet. As the diet becomes more Westernized, it is possible that we will see a proportionate rise in certain forms of cancer. One study of Japanese immigrant women living in San Francisco showed that they had twice the rate of breast cancer as their cousins living in Japan—no doubt due to a change in dietary habits.

### PEANUTS

The peanut agglutinin has also been found to contain a specific lectin sensitive to breast cancer cells, particularly the medullary form. The peanut lectin shows activity to a lesser degree against all other forms, including intraductal, lobular, and scirrhous breast cancers. This connection is probably true of other Type A–like cancers.

Eat fresh peanuts with the skins still on them (the skins, not the shells). Peanut butter is probably not a good source of the lectin, as the majority of commercial brands are too processed and homogenized.

### Amaranth

The grain amaranth contains a lectin that has a specific affinity to colon cancer cells. It programs the cancer cells to kill themselves, a process known as apoptosis.

### Mushrooms and Fava Beans

Commercial (silver dollar) mushrooms and fava beans contain lectins that react and suppress the T antigen. If you have a history of colon polyps, which are often a precancerous condition, you may want to increase your consumption of these foods. An amazing series of studies have shown that these lectins actually reverse many of the precancerous changes in the colon, reprogramming cells to change back to a more normal state.

### Lentils

The lectin found in common domestic brown or green lentils (*Lens culinaris*) shows a strong specific attraction for lobular, medullary, intraductal, and stromal forms of breast cancer and is likely to affect other A-like cancers.

### Lima Beans

Lima bean lectin is one of the most potent agglutinants of all Type A cells, cancerous or not. When you're healthy, lima beans will hurt you—so they shouldn't be part of a prevention strategy. However, if you are suffering from an A-like cancer, eat the lima beans. The lectin will agglutinate untold numbers of cancer cells. It will also destroy some perfectly innocent and upstanding Type A cells, but the exchange is worth it.

### Wheat Germ

Wheat germ agglutinin shows a great affinity for Type A cancers. It is concentrated in the seed coating of the wheat, the outer husk that is usually discarded. Unprocessed wheat bran will provide the most significant quantity of the lectin, although you can also use commercial wheat germ preparations.

SNAILS

If you're Type A or Type AB, order escargots the next time you dine at a fancy French restaurant. Consider it medicine packaged in a glamorous, delicious form. The edible snail, *Helix aspersa/pomatia*, is a powerful breast cancer agglutinin, capable of determining whether cancerous cells will metastasize to the lymph nodes.

Unless the thought of eating snails disgusts you (and really, they're quite delicious), what harm can it do? A colleague of mine from Italy once showed me a fifteenth-century manuscript that advised medieval physicians "to have the woman eat snails should she have crab-like scarring of the breast."

## Other Strategies

TAKE CARE OF YOUR LIVER AND COLON

Women should be aware that the liver and colon are two major sites where estrogens can be degraded—if their functions are disturbed, the levels of estrogen throughout the body can rise. Elevated estrogen activity can stimulate the growth of cancerous cells.

Adopt a high-fiber diet to increase the levels of butyrate in the colon wall cells. Butyrates, as you may recall, promote the normalization of tissue.

ANTIOXIDANTS

Vitamin antioxidants have been studied for breast cancer and have been shown to be not very effective in preventing the disease. Vitamin E and beta-carotenes don't deposit in high enough concentrations in breast tissue to effect positive change. Plant-based antioxidants do seem to make some difference but must be combined with supplemental sources of vitamin C to synergize for greatest effect.

Yellow onions contain very high levels of quercetin, an especially potent antioxidant. Quercetin has none of the estrogenizing activity of vitamin E and is hundreds of times stronger than vitamin antioxidants. It is available as a supplement in many health food stores.

Women with a risk factor for breast cancer who are considering or are on estrogen-replacement therapy should use phytoestrogens derived from natural products instead of synthetic estrogens. Plant-based estrogens contain high levels of estriol, a weaker form of the estrogen hormone than estradiol, which is manufactured synthetically. Estriol seems to lower your chances of developing breast cancer. The synthetics increase the risk. Tamoxifen, an estrogen-blocking drug prescribed to breast cancer patients with estrogen-sensitive breast tumors, is itself a weaker form of estrogen. Genistein is an estrogen-related compound found in the soybean lectin. This phytoestrogen inhibits angiogenesis, interfering with the production of new blood vessels needed to feed the growth of cancerous tumors.

### SPROUTED VEGETABLES

Sprouting vegetables unlock powerful medicines hidden within them. This is especially true if the vegetables are part of the cruciferous family, which when sprouted liberate large amounts of a powerful anticancer molecule known as sulforaphane. Sulforaphane has well-researched effects on DNA, encouraging its proper repair and controlling how genes are expressed in response to environmental stimulation.

### GENERAL PALLIATIVES

Exercise frequently. Get adequate rest. Have adequate creative expression in your life. Avoid known pollutants and pesticides. Eat your fruits and vegetables. Don't use antibiotics indiscriminately. If you get sick, allow your immune system to fight off the illness. You'll be much healthier if you do, rather than relying excessively on flu shots or antibiotics. They suppress your immune system's natural responses, which can be very powerful if given the chance.

### CASE HISTORY: ADVANCED BREAST CANCER
### JANE, AGE 50; BLOOD TYPE AB

When I first saw Jane in my office, she had already had a mastectomy and several rounds of chemotherapy for an infiltrating ductal breast cancer that extensively seeded into the lymph nodes. At the time of her initial diagnosis, Jane had two separate tumors on her left breast—one 4 centimeters and the other 1.5 centimeters. No one was holding out any great hope for her long-term survival.

I put Jane on the modified cancer diet for Type AB, with an emphasis on soy; I had her pneumovaxed; and I put her on the botanical protocol I use for Type As with breast cancer. Her tumor marker, CA15-3, which was 166 when she came in (normal is less than 10) dropped to 87 within three months and to 34 within four months of following my protocol. I recommended that she go see Georg Springer in Chicago to see if she could get into his vaccine study, which she did.

To this day all signs, including bone scans, look promising, although because Jane is a Type AB, I would be hesitant to pronounce her cured at this point. Only time will tell.

Cancer prevention and natural immune-system enhancement offer the brightest hope for the future. Genetic research is bringing us ever closer to being able to understand—perhaps someday even control—the cellular workings of these astounding machines that we call our bodies.

Cancer has long been among the most dreaded diseases of mankind. We seem powerless to protect ourselves and those we love from its clinging and relentless grip. Blood type analysis allows us a deeper understanding of our susceptibilities. By consciously examining our exposures to both environmental and dietary carcinogens and changing some of our lifestyle and food choices, we can minimize the effects of cell damage.

Blood type analysis also provides a way to enhance the ability of the immune system to search out and destroy cancerous and mutated cells while they are few in number. Cancer patients can use their knowledge of blood type to fully develop the capabilities of their immune systems to fight the disease. They can also gain a greater understanding of the mechanisms involved in the growth and spread of cancer.

The treatments for cancer are still far from perfect, although many people have been saved by the latest advances in therapy and scientific medical knowledge. For those of you with cancer and for those of you who have a family history of cancer, the advice is clear: Change your diet, change your attitudes, and start using antioxidant supplements. If you follow these suggestions you will be able to gain more control and a greater peace of mind. We all dread this horrible disease, but we can take positive action against it.

**FURTHER READING ABOUT YOUR BLOOD TYPE AND CANCER**

Three books in my Blood Type Diet series can give you more detailed information about your blood type and cancer:

- *Live Right 4 Your Type: The Individualized Prescription for Maximizing Health, Metabolism, and Vitality in Every Stage of Your Life*
- *Eat Right 4 Your Type Complete Blood Type Encyclopedia: The A–Z Reference Guide for the Blood Type Connection to Symptoms, Disease, Conditions, Vitamins, Supplements, Herbs, and Foods*
- *Cancer: Fight It with the Blood Type Diet*

EPILOGUE

# Individuals Evolving Together:

## *The Next Frontier*

The human journey began as the success story of one immune system—Type O. Not necessarily the first by molecular design, but certainly the most effective early survivor. It is an ineffable mystery as to precisely why Type A, the first molecular type, seemed to disappear, then resurrect itself as little as 40,000 years ago, but undoubtedly changes in diet, disease, location, and behavior exerted very strong influences. As those influences further evolved, different circumstances in specific parts of the world seemed to favor Type B. Finally, there is Type AB, not a true construct in a developmental sense, but rather the odd attribute only we humans possess of making a different blood type by combining two elemental ones.

We are always learning. Today, thanks to the pioneering work of the Human Genome Project, we are able to map the genetic structure of the human body—to name, gene by gene, chromosome by chromosome, the purpose of each living cell in the grand scheme of some master builder. Thus far, many breakthroughs have come in our understanding of the vast cellular networks of which we are composed—among them, the discovery of a large genetic architecture for breast cancer. Soon we will be able to control our genetic fates as never before.

*Should I take a multivitamin every day on the Blood Type Diet?*

If you are in good health and are following your Blood Type Diet, you shouldn't really need a supplement, although there are many possible exceptions. Pregnant women should supplement their diet with iron, calcium, and folic acid. Most women also need extra calcium—especially if their diet doesn't include many dairy foods.

Those engaged in heavy physical activity, people in stressful occupations, the elderly, those who are ill, heavy smokers—all should be on a supplementation program. More specific details are available in your individual Blood Type Diet.

*How important are herbs and herbal teas?*

The importance of herbs and herbal teas depends on your blood type. Type O responds well to soothing herbs, Type A to the more stimulating ones, and Type B does quite nicely without most of them. Type AB should follow the herbal protocols given for Type A, with the added proviso that Type AB shuns those herbs that both Type A and Type B are asked to avoid.

*Why are vegetable oils so limited on the Blood Type Diet? I thought all vegetable oils were good for you.*

What you've probably heard is advertisers hawking the news that vegetable oils have no cholesterol. Well, that's not news to anyone with even a modicum of knowledge about nutrition. Plants and vegetables do not manufacture cholesterol, which is found only in products derived from animals. Your cholesterol-free oil may have little else to recommend it.

Oils are very blood type specific, and you'll need to consult the recommendations for your type. I prefer to use olive oil as much as possible in cooking. I believe that olive oil has proven to be the most tolerated and beneficial of fats. As a monounsaturated oil it seems to have positive effects on the heart and arteries. There are many different blends of olive oil available. The finest quality is the extra-virgin grade. It is slightly greenish in color and almost odorless—although when gently heated, the perfume of the olives is sensational. Olive oil is usually cold-pressed rather than extracted using heat or chemicals. The less processed an oil is, the better its quality.

*Tofu seems like a very unappealing food. Must I eat it if I'm Type A?*

Many Type A and Type AB people are initially resistant to the idea that they make tofu a staple of their diets. Well, tofu is not a glamour food. I admit it. When I was an impoverished Type A college student, I ate tofu with vegetables and brown rice almost every day for years. It was cheap, but I actually liked it.

I think the real problem with tofu is the way it is usually displayed in the markets. Tofu—in soft or hard cakes—sits with its other tofu friends in a large plastic tub, immersed in cold water. Thankfully, tofu has grown more common as an ingredient in foods, and many restaurants regularly serve up delicious dishes whose main protein is tofu.

If you are going to use tofu, it is best cooked and combined with vegetables and strong flavors that you enjoy, such as garlic, ginger, and soy sauce. Tofu is a nutritionally complete food that is filling and extremely inexpensive. Type A take note: The path to your good health is paved with bean curd!

*I've never heard of many of the grains you mention. Where do I find out more?*

If you're looking for alternative grains, health food stores are a bonanza. In recent years, many ancient grains, largely forgotten, have been rediscovered and are now being produced. Examples of these are amaranth, a grain from Mexico, and spelt, a variation of wheat that seems to be free of the problems found with whole wheat. Try them! They're not bad. Spelt flour makes a hearty, chewy bread that is quite flavorful, while several interesting breakfast cereals are now being made with amaranth. Another alternative is to use sprouted-wheat breads, sometimes referred to as Manna or Essene bread, as the gluten lectins found principally in the seed coat are destroyed by the sprouting process. These breads spoil rapidly and are usually found in the refrigerator cases of health food stores. They are a live food, with many beneficial enzymes still intact. Beware of commercially produced sprouted wheat breads, as they usually have a minority of sprouted wheat and a majority of whole wheat in their formulas. Sprouted bread is somewhat sweet tasting, as the sprouting process also releases sugars, and it is moist and chewy. This bread makes wonderful toast.

*I'm Type A and I've been a runner for many years. Running seems to be a great way to reduce stress. I'm confused about your advice that I shouldn't exercise heavily.*

There is a great deal of evidence that your blood type informs your unique reaction to stress, and that Type A tends to do better with less intense exercise. My father observed this thousands of times in his 35 years studying the connection. However, there is much we don't yet know, so I would hesitate to say absolutely that you shouldn't run.

I would ask you to reevaluate your health and energy levels. I often have patients who say things like, "I've always been a runner," or "I've always eaten chicken," as if that were all the proof they needed that an activity or a food was beneficial. Often, these very people are suffering from an assortment of physical problems and stresses that they've never thought to associate with specific activities or foods. You may be a Type A with a twist—one who thrives on intense physical activity—or you may discover that you're running on empty.

*Should I avoid genetically engineered (GMO) food?*

Yes! Genetic engineering often involves moving lectin molecules from one species to another. Because lectins are the molecules that interact with our blood types, an okay food can easily become one to avoid. Currently, because GMO content is not required to be listed on the food label, the only way to safely avoid GMO foods is to choose organic.

*Why should all blood types avoid pork?*

Hog is very A-like immunologically, which makes it an avoid food if you happen to have antibodies to the Blood Type A antigen, like Type B and Type O do. Paradoxically, hog also has an antibody (isohemagglutinin) in its tissues that reacts to the A antigen, so it should be avoided for this reason by Type A and Type AB as well. A surprising number of people carry antibodies in their blood type to pork products.

*You mentioned that most Native Americans are Type O. I was wondering (being a Type O) about the use of corn because many tribes have used that as a staple.*

Corn is a sacred food in many Native American cultures. Unfortunately, that doesn't make it any better as a health choice! A good example of the effect in adding corn into the diet of Type O Native Americans can be observed in the bone remains of the Indiana Mound Building cultures. We can exactly trace the introduction of corn into their diet after their long history as hunter-gatherers, by the marked change in their bone structure. Before corn became a staple, the bones show little arthritis or thinning; after corn was introduced, bone deformation began, including major changes to the teeth structure and jaw (periodontal disease). In addition, maize stimulates a very rapid and powerful glycemic response, so it may be that the switch to a maize-based diet from a hunter-gatherer way of life may have been responsible for a precipitous increase in diabetes. If corn lectins are problematic for Type O, they are even more serious as a hemagglutinin in Type B and Type AB individuals.

*Aside from blood type principles, from a general health standpoint, are there any food choice tips?*

Organic produce, organic dairy, and free-range meats are recommended. Genetically altered foods (which includes virtually all nonorganic soybeans), hydrogenated oils (margarine), partially hydrogenated oils, and artificial additives (sweeteners, colors, aromas, and flavors) should be avoided. Smoked and fried foods are not recommended. Oils should be purchased and stored in lightproof containers and preferably refrigerated after opening. White flour and sugars should be eaten rarely, if at all. MSG should not be used. Avoid aluminum cookery (it can contaminate your food with aluminum), and microwaves (they change the molecular structure of foods in unknown ways) for cooking.

*One of my friends sees a naturopathic doctor who claims that naturopathic philosophy is based exclusively on vegetarian diets.*

This association is so ingrained in the belief systems of some individuals that to even suggest that appropriate consumption of animal foods might actually enhance some individuals' health places me somewhere between public enemy number one and the devil in the eyes of several of my critics. Furthermore, veganism, which rejects all animal-based foods, even eggs and dairy, has been gaining popularity at a rapid pace—and that trend seems particularly prominent among millennials.

Often a good question to ask is, what does the evidence show? Naturopathic medicine developed from the water cure movement of Europe. Theodor Hahn is credited as being the first to integrate vegetarian dietary principles into the water cure movement. He was convinced that a meat-free diet would prolong life. In fact he was so convinced of the value of a vegetarian diet that he spent a great deal of his professional life writing books and pamphlets on the subject and was the editor of a magazine called the *Vegetarian*. He died of colon cancer at the age of 59. The point is, before you make a decision to adopt a particular diet, understand your reasons—apart from vague claims—and look at the evidence. If your goal is a long and healthy life, don't base your choices on someone's philosophy, but on what will help you reach that goal. I like a quote from the Talmud, an ancient rabbinical text, that pretty much sums it up: "Feed me in ways that are convenient for me."

*How can it be that wheat isn't good for anyone? Hasn't it been a staple in the human diet for thousands of years?*

Wheat, as we know it today, is not the same as it was when humans first started eating it. The genetics of wheat show that its development has been very complex. Today's grain is derived from three groups of wheat. Through natural crossings, mutations, and natural selection, these have evolved into all the many varieties of wheat grown worldwide.

In essence, the hard wheat that we eat nowadays has a protein content as high as 13 percent, versus the more ancient wheats, which had a protein content of, at most, about 2 percent. Increasing the protein content has had the effect of making wheat a viable source of protein for many people around the world, but this has also increased the allergenic (gliadin-, gluten-, and lectin-containing), proinflammatory, and metabolic-blocking portions of the plant almost sevenfold.

Aside from the underinvestigated metabolic effects of wheat lectin, classic hypersensitivity to wheat is found in many infants and adults. Reactions are often localized in the GI tract. In a study of asthma patients, 46 percent of children and 34 percent of adults were found to have immunoglobulin E (IgE) to wheat as tested by Pharmacia CAP System. In another study, specificity for wheat allergen using the same system was 98 percent. Wheat allergy was found to cause a persistent food hypersensitivity in 75 percent of atopic dermatitis patients. In 102 children who had grass pollen allergies, 12 percent were found to be allergic to wheat.

*I appear to be allergic or reactive to a highly beneficial food. What do I do?*

Don't eat it. In the event that your body has been altered by drugs, surgery, or disease, you may have different tolerances for food. The best thing to do in this situation is avoid the allergy-causing food and the other avoid foods for your blood type. Choose as many beneficial and neutral foods as possible. This sensitivity may change over time.

*Are there any healthy sugars or sweeteners for my blood type?*

Refined sugar is considered as addictive as a drug and potentially as detrimental to your health. Yet, according to the U.S. Department of Agriculture, the average American consumes between 150 and 170 pounds of refined sugar each year! It is clear that collectively we have a serious habit to kick. Sure, there are plenty of sugar-free sweetener alternatives on the market, but those chemically created artificial sweeteners are even more toxic than refined sugar. Ending your sugar addiction doesn't mean that you have to stop enjoying a hint of sweetness—it just requires that you find healthier alternatives. Fortunately, there are some all-natural, blood-type-friendly options.

Agave nectar is a honey-like sweetener made from the sap found in the core of the agave plant. It's sweeter than table sugar, so you can use less to get the same results, while at the same time boosting your recommended daily allowance of vitamins and minerals: It has trace amounts of calcium, iron, potassium, and magnesium. Agave nectar also has a lower glycemic index than table sugar, so it won't cause a spike in blood sugar levels. It's neutral for all blood types and both secretors and non-secretors.

Raw organic local honey contains trace amounts of niacin, riboflavin, thiamin, vitamin $B_6$, and free-radical-fighting antioxidants, and, some studies show, may help alleviate seasonal allergies. If you're trying to lose weight, there's good news for you; honey's low glycemic index helps keep sugar levels in check, and it's 50 percent sweeter than refined sugar, so you'll be satisfied with less. It's neutral for all blood type secretors, but should be avoided by Type O and Type AB non-secretors.

Pure maple syrup can be used as a sugar substitute in baking. Research shows that maple syrup also has some health benefits, including promoting cardiovascular health and boosting the immune system. It's neutral for all blood type secretors but should be avoided by Type O and Type AB non-secretors.

Molasses is the product of the refining of sugar cane and sugar beets; the juice squeezed from these plants is boiled to a syrupy mixture from which sugar crystals are extracted. The remaining brownish-black liquid is molasses. Molasses is a popular sweetener in baking and can also be used as a syrup on pancakes and waffles. Its health benefits include a high iron content as well as vitamin $B_6$, magnesium, calcium, and more antioxidants than any other natural sweetener. It's beneficial for Type A secretors and neutral for all the other blood types.

Stevia is the powdered extract of the plant *Stevia rebaudiana*, an herb indigenous to Paraguay and Brazil. While this zero-calorie sugar substitute tastes just like table sugar, it won't cause a spike in blood sugar levels. When using stevia, note that it is 200 to 400 times sweeter than sugar and you should use far less when baking or stirring it into coffee or tea. Health benefits include phytochemical compounds that help control blood sugar, cholesterol, and blood pressure. It's neutral for most blood types, but should be avoided by Type B secretors and Type O non-secretors.

APPENDIX D

# Glossary of Terms

ABO BLOOD GROUP SYSTEM: THE MOST IMPORTANT OF THE BLOOD-TYPING systems, the ABO blood group is the determinant for transfusion reactions and organ transplantation. Unlike the other blood-typing systems, the ABO blood types have far-ranging significance other than transfusion or transplantation, including the determination of many of the digestive and immunological characteristics of the body. The ABO blood group is made up of four blood types: O, A, B, and AB. Type O has no true antigen but carries antibodies to both A and B blood. Type A and Type B carry the antigen named for their blood type and make antibodies to each other. Type AB does not manufacture any antibodies to other blood types because it has both A and B antigens. Anthropologists use the ABO blood types extensively as a guide to the development of early peoples. Many diseases—especially digestive disorders, cancer, and infection—express preferences among the ABO blood types.

*Agglutinate:* Derived from the Latin word for "to glue." The process by which cells are made to adhere to one another, usually through the actions of an agglutinin, such as an antibody or a lectin. Certain viruses and bacteria also are capable of agglutinating blood cells. Many agglutinins, particularly food lectins, are blood type specific. Certain foods clump only the cells of one blood type but do not react with the cells of another type.

*Allele:* An alternative form of a gene, such as the blood type alleles, A, B and O.

*Anthropology:* The study of humankind in relation to distribution, origin, and classification. Anthropologists study human evolution, human physical characteristics, the relationships among ethnic groups, the interaction between the environment and society, and ancient and modern culture. ABO blood types have been extensively used by anthropologists in the study of early human populations.

*Antibody:* A class of chemicals, called the immunoglobulins, made by the cells of the immune system to specifically tag or identify foreign material within the body of the host. Antibodies combine with specific markers—antigens—found on viruses, bacteria, or other toxins and agglutinate them. The immune system is capable of manufacturing millions of different antibodies against a wide variety of potential invaders. Individuals of Type O, Type A, or Type B blood carry antibodies to other blood types. Type AB, the universal recipient, manufactures no antibodies to other types.

*Antigen:* Any chemical that causes the immune system to generate an antibody in response to it. The chemical markers that determine blood type are considered blood type antigens because other blood types may carry antibodies to them. Antigens are commonly found on the surface of germs, and are used by the immune system to detect foreign material. Specialized antigens are often made by cancer cells and are called tumor antigens. Many germs and cancer antigens are clever impersonators that can mimic the blood type of the host in an effort to escape detection by the immune system.

*Antioxidants:* Vitamins that are believed to strengthen the immune system and prevent cancer by fighting off toxic compounds (called free radicals) that attack cells. Vitamins C and E and beta-carotene are believed to be the most powerful antioxidants.

*Cro-Magnon:* The first truly modern human. Cro-Magnon migrated extensively from Africa into Europe and Asia. A master hunter, Cro-Magnon led a largely hunter-gatherer existence. Most of the digestive characteristics of people with Type O blood are derived from Cro-Magnon.

*Differentiation:* The cellular process by which cells develop their specialized characteristics and functions. Differentiation is controlled by the genetic machinery of the cell. Cancer cells, which often have defective genes, usually de-evolve and lose many of the characteristics of a normal cell, often reverting to earlier embryologic forms long repressed since early development.

*Gene:* A component of the cell that controls the transmission of hereditary characteristics by specifying the construction of a particular protein or enzyme. Genes are composed of long chains of deoxyribonucleic acid (DNA) contained in the chromosomes of the cell nucleus.

*Indo-European:* An early white people who migrated westward to Europe from their original homelands in Asia and the Middle East in 7,000 to 3,500 B.C.E. The Indo-Europeans were probably the progenitors for Type A blood in western Europe.

*Ketosis:* A state that is achieved with a high-protein, low-carbohydrate diet. The high-protein diets of our early Type O ancestors forced the burning of fat for energy and the production of ketones—a sign of rapid metabolic activity. The state of ketosis allowed early humans to maintain high energy, metabolic efficiency, and physical strength—all qualities needed for hunting game.

*Lectin:* Any compound, usually a protein, found in nature that can interact with surface antigens found on the body's cells, causing them to agglutinate. Lectins are often found in common foods, and many of them are blood type specific. Because cancer cells often manufacture copious amounts of antigens on their surface, many lectins will agglutinate them in preference to normal cells.

*Microbiome:* The collection of microorganisms that make up your internal ecosystem. The health of the microbiome depends on an abundance of healthy bacteria.

*Mucus:* Secretions manufactured by specialized tissues, called mucous membranes, which are used to lubricate and protect the delicate internal linings of the body. Mucus contains antibodies to protect against germs. In secretors, large amounts of blood type antigens are secreted in mucus, which serves to filter out bacteria, fungi, and parasites with opposing blood type characteristics.

*Naturopathic doctor (ND):* A physician trained in natural healing methods. Naturopathic doctors receive four-year postgraduate training at an accredited college or university, and function as primary-care providers.

*Neolithic:* The period of early human development characterized by the development of agriculture and the use of pottery and polished tools. The radical change in human lifestyle, from the previous hunter-gatherer existence, probably was a major stimulus to the development of Blood Type A.

*Panhemagglutinins:* Lectins that agglutinate all blood types. An example is the tomato lectin.

*Polymorphism:* Literally means "many shapes." A polymorphism is any physical manifestation within a species of living organisms that is variable through genetic influence. The blood types are a well-known polymorphism.

*Phytochemical:* Any natural product with specific health applications. Most phytochemicals are traditional herbs and plants.

*Triglycerides:* The body's fat stores, also contained in the bloodstream. High triglycerides, or high blood fats, are considered a risk for heart disease.

APPENDIX E

# Notes on the Anthropology of Blood Type

ANTHROPOLOGY IS THE STUDY OF HUMAN DEVELOPMENT AND DIFFERences, both cultural and biological. For our purposes, we can look at the way the field is divided into two categories: cultural anthropology, which looks at the manifestations of culture, such as language and ritual, and biological anthropology, the study of the evolutionary biology of our species, *Homo sapiens*. Biological anthropologists attempt to trace human historical development through hard scientific methods, such as examining the blood types. A central task in biological anthropology has been to document the sequence of how the human line evolved from early nonhuman primate ancestors. The use of blood types to study early societies has been termed paleoserology, the study of ancient blood.

Biological anthropology is also concerned with how humans adapted to environmental pressures. Traditional biological anthropology relied heavily on the measuring of skull shape, stature, and other physical characteristics. Blood type became a powerful tool for this type of analysis in the 1950s, as emphasis shifted to genetic characteristics, such as blood types and other genetic markers. A. E. Mourant, a physician and anthropologist, published two key works, *Blood Groups and Diseases* (1978) and *Blood Relations: Blood Groups and Anthropology* (1983), that collected much of the available material on the subject.

In addition to Mourant, I've used a variety of other source material for this appendix, including earlier anthropology sources such as William Boyd's *Genetics and the Races of Man* (1950), and a series of studies that were published in various journals of forensic medicine from 1920 to 1945.

It is possible to map the occurrence of the various blood groups in ancient populations by blood typing grave exhumations. Small amounts of blood type materials can be reconstituted from the remains and the blood type determined. By studying the blood types of human populations, anthropologists gain information about that population's local history, movement, intermarriage, and diversification.

Many national and ethnic groups have unique blood type distributions. In certain more isolated cultures, a clear majority of one blood type over another can still be seen. In other societies, it may be more evenly distributed. In the United States, for example, the equal rates of Type O and Type A blood reflect masses of immigration.

The United States also has a higher percentage of Blood Type B than the western European countries, which probably reflects the influx of more eastern nationalities.

For the purpose of this analysis, we can divide humankind into two basic clusters—Ethiopian and Palearctic. The Palearctic can be further broken down to Mongolians and Caucasians, although most people lie somewhere in between. Each race is physically characterized by its environment and occupies distinct geographic areas. Ethiopians, probably the oldest race, are dark-skinned Africans, inhabiting the southern third of Arabia and sub-Saharan Africa. The Palearctic region is made up of Africa north of the Sahara; Europe; and most of Asia, including India, Southeast Asia, and southern China but with the exception of southern Arabia.

The roughest guesswork places the beginnings of human migration from Africa to Asia at about 1 million years ago. In Asia, most likely, the modern *Homo sapiens* species split from a trunk of the ancestral Ethiopians into the Caucasians and Mongolians, but we know almost nothing about when or why it occurred.

Each of the basic races has its own homeland—a geographic area where it is preeminent. The Ethiopian homeland was Africa; the Caucasian, Europe and northern Asia; and the Mongolian, central and southern Asia. There may be more physical differences between Africans and the other races, but the blood type differences between Caucasians and Mongolians are more clear-cut—a good reason to reexamine racial stereotypes.

Although we trace the numerical predominance and ascent of Type O blood back to early prehistory, it still remains a very workable chemistry, largely because of its simplicity and the fact that animal protein diets still account for a great portion of the world's current food intake.

The first attempt at using blood type to describe ethnic and nationality characteristics was undertaken by a husband-and-wife team of physicians, the Hirszfelds, in 1918. During World War I both had served as doctors in the Allied armies that had concentrated in the area of Salonika, Greece. Working with a multinational force, the Hirszfelds systematically blood-typed large numbers of refugees of different ethnic backgrounds, also recording their race and nationality. Each group contained at least five hundred subjects.

The Hirszfelds found, for example, that the rate of Blood Type B ranged from a low of 7.2 percent of the population of English subjects to a high of 41.2 percent in Indians, and that western Europeans in general had a lower incidence of Type B than Balkan Slavs, who had a lower incidence than Russians, Turks, and Jews, who again had a lower occurrence than Vietnamese and Indians. The distribution of Blood Type AB essentially followed the same pattern, with a low of 3 to 5 percent in western Europeans and a high of 8.5 percent in Indians.

In subcontinental India, Type AB makes up 8.5 percent of the population—remarkably high for a blood type that typically averages between 2 and 5 percent worldwide. This prevalence of Type AB is probably due to subcontinental India's location as an invasion route between the conquered lands to the west and the Mongolian homelands to the east.

Blood Type O and Type A were essentially the reverse of Type B and Type AB. The percentage of Type A remained fairly consistent (40 percent) among Europeans, Balkan Slavs, and Arabs, while being quite low in West Africans, Vietnamese, and Indians. About 46 percent of the English population tested were Type O, which accounted for only 31.3 percent of the Indians tested.

Modern analysis (largely the result of records kept by blood banks), encompasses the blood types of more than 20 million individuals from around the world. Yet these large numbers can do no more than confirm the original observations of the Hirszfelds. No scientific journals saw fit to publish their material at that time. For a while, the Hirszfelds' study languished in an obscure anthropology journal; for more than 30 years this fascinating and important work was overlooked.

Apparently, there was little interest in using this knowledge of the blood types as an anthropological probe into the history of humanity.

Recent work by Dr. Luigi Cavalli-Sforza at Stanford University has tracked the genetic movement of ancient humans, using even more sophisticated methods based on the new DNA technology. Many of his findings have confirmed the earlier observations of Mourant, the Hirszfelds, Snyder, and Boyd concerning the distribution of blood types worldwide.

APPENDIX F

# The Blood Type Support Community

## Discover Your Blood Type

It is difficult to begin a diet based on blood type if you are not aware of your own type. In Europe, blood type is something almost everyone knows, but here in the United States, unless we need a transfusion, we can go our entire lives without knowing what blood type we are. What follow are several simple ways to find out your blood type:

1. Donate blood. Not only are you providing a critical service to the community but this is a free and simple way to find out what blood type you are. To find your local donation center, visit the American Red Cross website's Give Blood page (redcrossblood.org).
2. Purchase a blood-typing kit from D'Adamo Personalized Nutrition (4yourtype.com), under "Books and Tests." The kit is inexpensive and simple to do in your own home.
3. Next time you visit your doctor for a blood workup, ask him or her to add blood typing to the blood test protocol.

## Secretor Status

If you do not know your secretor status and want to further refine your personalized profile, you can purchase a Secretor Status Collection Kit from D'Adamo Personalized Nutrition (4yourtype.com).

## Center of Excellence in Generative Medicine

The Center of Excellence in Generative Medicine (COEGM) is a collaboration between Peter D'Adamo and the University of Bridgeport (UB) to create a frontiers-focused biomedical initiative without parallel in any other medical school. The COEGM combines patient care, clinical research, and hands-on teaching opportunities for students of the university's health sciences program. It is also home to Dr. D'Adamo's clinical practice and uses his state-of-the-art bioinformatic software programs like SWAMI GenoType and Opus23. For information and appointments for either private practice patients or clinic-shift patients, please contact the center at:

Center of Excellence in Generative Medicine
115 Broad Street
Bridgeport, CT 06604
203-366-0526
generativemedicine.org

## For All Things Peter D'Adamo—dadamo.com

One of the longest-running websites on the Internet, dadamo.com is the home page for the community of "netizens" who follow the work of Dr. Peter D'Adamo. This easy-to-navigate site is chock-full of helpful tools, blogs, and one of the warmest, most welcoming chat forums to be found. Newbies are welcome to this moderated, family-friendly community.

## D'Adamo Personalized Nutrition—North American Pharmacal, Inc.

For information on the Blood Type Diet, individualized supplements, and testing kits, please contact Dr. D'Adamo at:

D'Adamo Personalized Nutrition
North American Pharmacal, Inc.